AN ATLAS OF VULVAL DISEASE

An Atlas of Vulval Disease
A Combined Dermatological, Gynaecological and Venereological Approach

Michèle Leibowitch MD
Professor of Dermatology
Hôpital Tarnier, Paris, France

Richard Staughton MA, FRCP
Consultant Dermatologist
Chelsea and Westminster Hospital, London, UK

Sallie Neill MRCP
Consultant Dermatologist
St Peter's Hospital, Chertsey, Surrey; and
St John's Dermatology Centre, St Thomas's Hospital, London, UK

Simon Barton BSc, MD, MRCOG
Consultant Physician in Genito-Urinary Medicine
Chelsea and Westminster Hospital, London, UK

Roger Marwood MSc, FRCOG
Consultant Gynaecologist and Obstetrician
Chelsea and Westminster Hospital, London, UK

MARTIN DUNITZ

© Martin Dunitz Ltd 1995, 1997

First published in 1995 by
Martin Dunitz Ltd, The Livery House,
7–9 Pratt Street, London NW1 0AE

Second edition 1997

A CIP catalogue record for this title is available
from the British Library.

ISBN 1–85317–431–9

Composition by Scribe Design, Gillingham, Kent
Printed and bound in Singapore by
Kyodo Printing Co (S'pore) Pte Ltd

Contents

To
R.B.
C.P.M.S.
M.J.S.
V.A.B.
S.C.M.

Preface

This atlas has been compiled by specialists in dermatology, genito-urinary medicine, gynaecology and pathology.

The diagnosis and management of vulval dermatoses requires such a multidisciplinary approach and the importance of this has been amply demonstrated by the evolution of combined clinics. Too often in the past, complex dermatological conditions have been seen and managed by specialists inexperienced in such disorders, resulting in inappropriate treatment. Perhaps the worst example of this is the unfortunate patient who is subjected to the physical and psychological trauma of a vulvectomy and who is still not cured of her condition. The combined clinic is, therefore, ideal in that a woman will have all aspects of her disease considered and be offered the best therapeutic advice. In addition, there are the major advantages of improving education and dissemination of information across the specialties for both staff in training and senior staff alike.

A combined clinic was established at the Westminster Hospital in 1983 with Roger de Vere (Gynaecologist), Titus Oates (Genito-urinary specialist) and Richard Staughton (Dermatologist). This clinic forged strong links between the three departments, which still exist today, despite the retirements of both Roger de Vere and Titus Oates, who have been replaced by Roger Marwood and Simon Barton. The junior staff in the different specialties have exposure to the clinic in their training, very important for future practice. The number of patients seen in the clinic is growing rapidly every year as our hospital colleagues and family practitioners now recognize the great need for such a clinic. The recent founding of a European college for the study of vulvo-vaginal disease recognizes this need and should provide a good local forum for the dissemination of knowledge. The Health Service reforms in the UK do not adequately address the funding of multi-disciplinary clinics. This is a major error, and the authors hope that this problem will be rectified in the not-too-distant future.

Vulval disease in many societies can be the subject of unnecessary and exaggerated shame and embarrassment, hence their frequency and importance have been underestimated. Many women with symptoms delay for several years attending a physician because of fears about the source of the condition and the examinations which might be necessary to investigate it. It is the duty of physicians to do everything possible in their practice to minimize this understandable embarrassment and to promote such practice amongst other doctors.

We hope, therefore, that the wider dissemination that may be available to this economical atlas will increase the understanding of vulval disease and benefit the increasing numbers of women presenting with vulval dermatoses.

Acknowledgements

Our French colleagues at Hôpital Tarnier, under the guidance of Professor Jean Hewitt, formed one of the first combined clinics in 1970, gathering together a team of Dermato-venereologists, Gynaecologists and Pathologists. They have had a great influence on our practice and we have profited greatly from close collaboration with them. Their definitive text *Maladies de la vulve* published in 1987 (Jean Hewitt, Monique Pelisse and Bernard Paniel, Medisi-McGraw-Hill) and Marjorie Ridley's *The Vulva* (first edn, 1988, Churchill Livingstone) have been our constant sources of reference. It was, therefore, eminently appropriate that in preparing this atlas we should have enlisted the unrivalled experience of Professor Michèle Leibowitch, herself a Dermatologist and Pathologist and a member of the Tarnier team, whose knowledge and experience of the subject was invaluable. The majority of the histological illustrations in the atlas are also French, and we are extremely grateful to all our colleagues at the Hôpital Tarnier for their co-operation, encouragement and friendship over the years.

All who seek to treat patients with vulval disease have been inspired by the pioneers, Dr Hugh Wallace in London and Professor Jean Hewitt in Paris. Since their deaths, Dr Marjorie Ridley and Dr Monique Pelisse have replaced them as the great sources of clinical knowledge and experience to whom we have gratefully turned over the years.

We thank our very many colleagues who have contributed so generously with advice and photographic material for this atlas, especially Prof B Paniel, Mr R D de Vere, Mr V R Tindall, Drs S J Adams, A C Branfoot, C K Bridgett, C B Bunker, I Lindsey, D A Hawkins, A G Lawrence, C N Mallinson, S Mayou, M Moyal Barraco, M Pelisse and P L Samarasinghe.

We thank our electronic scribe Jennifer Fell for coping so well with five authors and bilingual dictaphonics. Alison Campbell, Rosemary Allen and Martin Dunitz have been kindly and patient publishers, and Kevin Marks produced the marvellous artwork.

Those at home who have tolerated our invasions and migrations: we salute you.

1 Anatomy of the vulva and classification of disease

Anatomy

The vulva is the collective term used to describe the female external genitalia. It includes the mons pubis anteriorly, the labia majora laterally enclosing the bilateral labia minora, the clitoris, clitoral hood and is bounded posteriorly by the posterior labial commissure. The innermost part is the vulval vestibule into which opens the urethra and vagina.

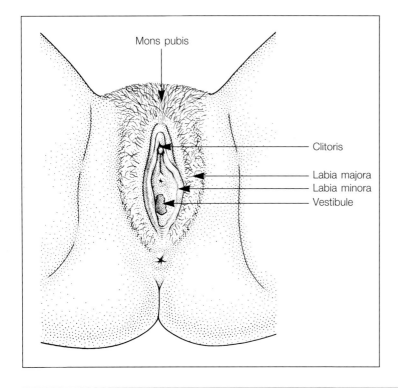

Figure 1.1

The vulva is comprised of the labia majora, the labia minora, clitoris, vestibule and mons pubis.

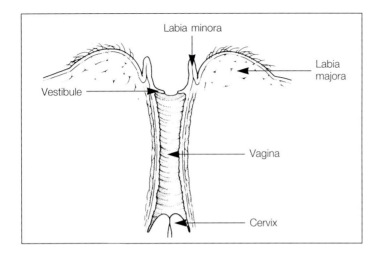

Figure 1.2
Diagrammatic section along the
axis of the vagina.

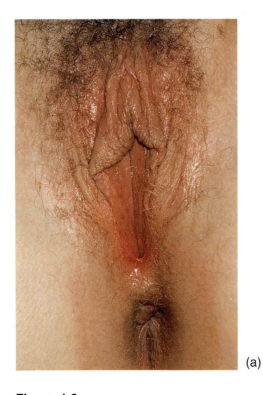

(a)

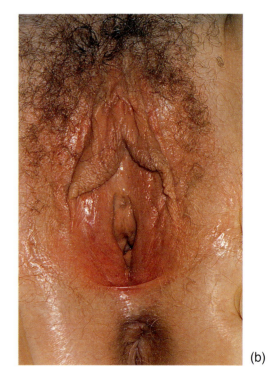

(b)

Figure 1.3
(a) The normal adult vulva. (b) The same vulva,
with the labia majora held apart, shows
vestibule and labia minora.

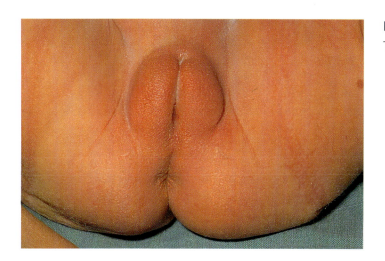

Figure 1.4
The vulva at birth.

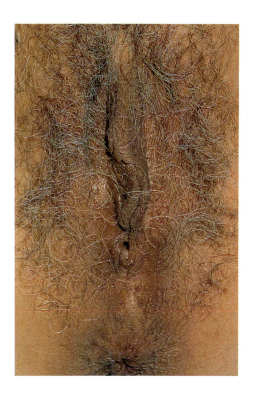

Figure 1.5
The adult vulva: black woman.

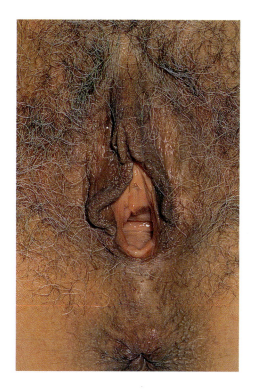

Figure 1.6
The adult vulva. Dermatoses in black skin may cause difficulties in diagnosis.

Micro-anatomy of the vulva

The various regions of the vulva bear different
appendages. The labia majora have a full
complement of adnexal structures, with hair follicles, and sebaceous, eccrine and apocrine
glands. The labia minora, like the areola, are
hairless but possess sebaceous glands. The
vestibule bears no pilosebaceous units.

The labia majora and minora have a cornified
stratified squamous epithelium. In the vestibule,
the squamous epithelium is non-cornified and
shows pale, heavily glycogenated suprabasal
cells. The vagina is likewise non-cornified but
even richer in glycogenated cells.

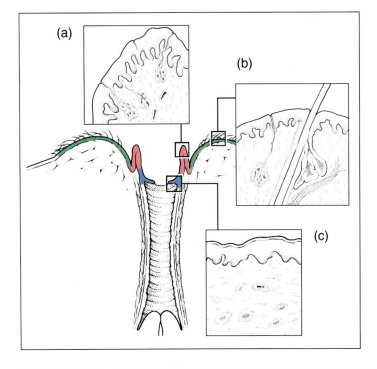

Figure 1.7

Comparison of epithelia at different
anatomical sites of the vulva.
(a) Labia minora; (b) labia majora;
(c) vestibule.

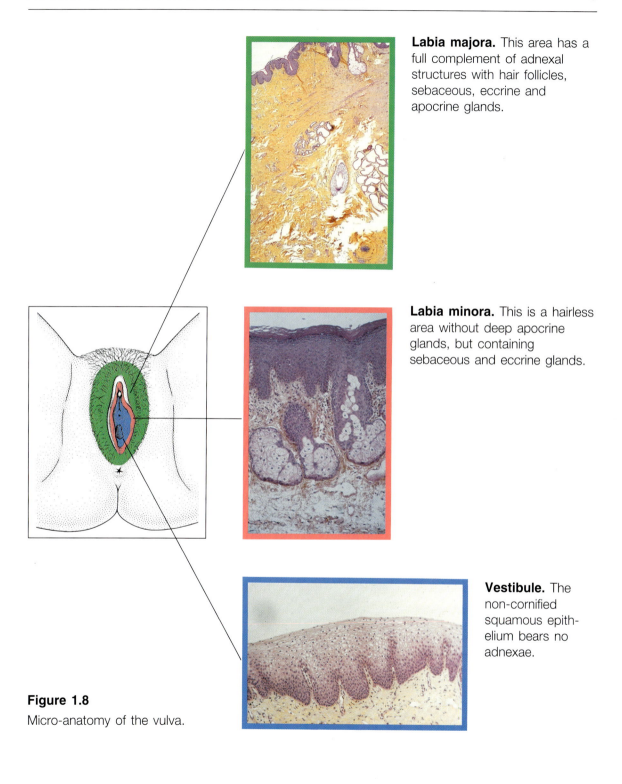

Labia majora. This area has a full complement of adnexal structures with hair follicles, sebaceous, eccrine and apocrine glands.

Labia minora. This is a hairless area without deep apocrine glands, but containing sebaceous and eccrine glands.

Vestibule. The non-cornified squamous epithelium bears no adnexae.

Figure 1.8
Micro-anatomy of the vulva.

Classification of disease

It is beyond the scope of this book to discuss the classification of vulval diseases in depth, particularly as this is currently being reconsidered. The classification recommended by the International Society for the Study of Vulvar Disease (ISSVD) and the International Society of Gynecological Pathologists (ISGP) in 1986, which is the most recent, is given in Table 1.1.

It has now been recommended that certain terms should no longer be used as a diagnosis:

- *Kraurosis vulvae*—this is now known to be lichen sclerosus.
- *Leucoplakia*—this is a descriptive term, meaning white plaque, and can now only be used as a clinical term. It is not a histopathological diagnosis.
- *Dystrophy*—the use of this term has been completely discontinued.

Table 1.1 Classification of vulval diseases

Benign
1. Lichen sclerosus
2. Squamous cell hyperplasia
3. Other dermatoses – e.g. psoriasis, lichen planus, etc.

Malignant
  Squamous
  VIN I   Atypia lower 1/3 epidermis
  VIN II   Atypia > 1/3 < 2/3 epidermis
  VIN III   Atypia > 2/3 or full thickness
  Non-squamous
    Paget's disease
    Malignant melanoma

2 Examination of the vulva

Equipment and specimen taking

Some authorities use a colposcope to examine external genitalia, but we find good lighting and a ×4 lens more than adequate for most cases. More commonly, it is used for directed biopsies of atypical areas and to follow direction of treatments such as cryotherapy and/or laser therapy.

A specimen from the lateral or posterior vaginal walls is appropriate for providing material for Gram staining and for culture for fungi and protozoal infections, as well as for the diagnosis of bacterial vaginosis.

Specimens from the endocervix can be used for diagnostic tests, for example for the detection of *Neisseia gonorrhoeae*, and *Chlamydia trachomatis.*

Urethral specimens can be taken as urethral secretions add to the sensitivity of the diagnosis of gonorrhoea. In women who have had a

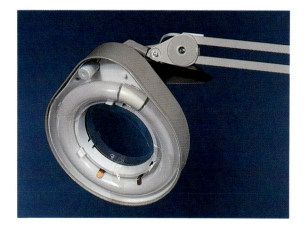

Figure 2.1
Examination light.

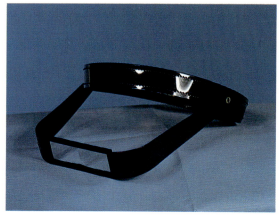

Figure 2.2
Head-worn magnifying loop.

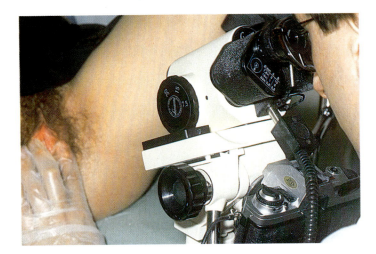

Figure 2.3
Colposcope.

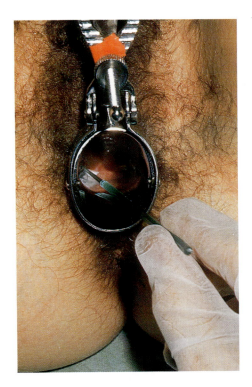

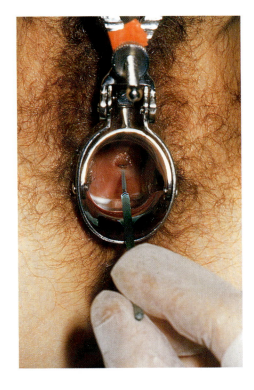

Figure 2.4
Taking a high vaginal swab from the lateral
vaginal wall.

Figure 2.5
Taking a specimen from the endocervix.

hysterectomy, gonococcal and chlamydial urethral infection have been described, and this area should be sampled along with the vaginal fornix and the anogenital skin.

Examination

Genital examination, both internal and external, is carried out in the presence of a trained chaperone to place the patient at maximum ease and to ensure the correct handling of specimens taken for the laboratory. In addition, procedures such as warming the speculum and keeping the patient's abdomen covered with a sheet or blanket can facilitate comfortable examination.

A systematic approach is required in order not to miss physical signs. It should start with a general view of the vulva, looking at the skin and hairs of the mons pubis and labia majora.

1. *General view*
   a. Hairs: i. Distribution and extent (e.g. alopecia areata, evidence of virilization)
                  ii. Quality and condition (e.g. colour, broken hairs from friction)
                  iii. Infestation.
   b. Skin colour: i. Pigmentary disturbance (e.g. vitiligo)
                   ii. Inflammation present or absent.

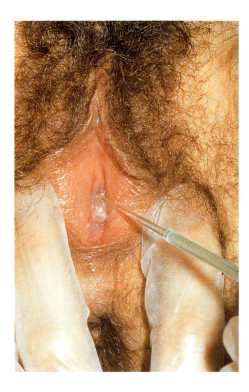

Figure 2.6
Taking a urethral specimen.

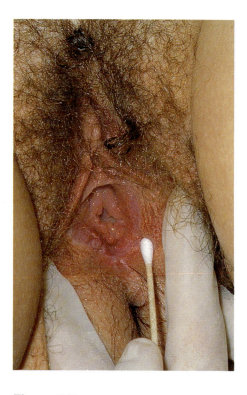

Figure 2.7
Palpation with cotton-tipped swab.

c. Skin texture: Abnormal thickness (e.g. lichenification or atrophy).
d. Skin surface: i. Integrity
                 ii. Excoriation
                 iii. Erosions.
e. Palpation: Tenderness or underlying masses (e.g. cysts).

2. *Labia minora*
   a. Presence or absence
   b. Developmental abnormality.

3. *Clitoral area*
   a. Hood
   b. Clitoris — normal size and surface.

4. *Vestibule*
   a. Urethral opening
   b. Vaginal aperture
   c. Epithelial surface — colour, texture and palpation with cotton-tipped swab.

5. *Perianal area*
   An examination of the vulva is not complete without an inspection of the whole perineum, including the perianal skin (embryologically derived from the cloaca).

Biopsy of the vulva

This is a simple procedure requiring a local anaesthetic and should be performed as an outpatient procedure, taking some 15 minutes. A punch biopsy is all that is usually needed, using either a 4 or 6 mm dermatopunch. It is important to state the exact site that is biopsied in the vulva, as the histology will differ according to what area is sampled.

Indications for biopsy include:

1. Difficulty in establishing a clinical diagnosis.
2. All blistering disorders: separate punch biopsy for immunofluorescence should be taken and placed in special transport media.

3. All pigmented lesions.
4. Inflammatory lesions that do not respond as expected to anti-inflammatory drugs in order to exclude neoplasia.
5. Persistently erosive lesions.

Procedure

1. Ten minutes before the biopsy an application of local anaesthetic cream (e.g. lignocaine plus prilocaine or lignocaine gel), from the

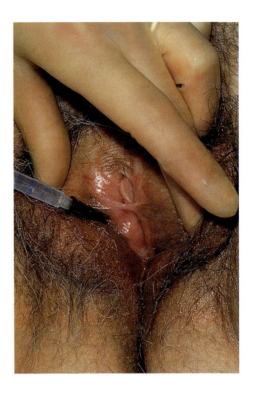

Figure 2.8
Instillation of plain lignocaine, 1%.

interlabial sulcus inwards, will blunt the pain of injection of local anaesthetic.

2. The area is cleaned with diluted chlorhexidine antiseptic.
3. Plain lignocaine (1%), with or without adrenaline, is instilled with a fine needle.
4. Surgical procedure:
   a. *Punch biopsy*—a 4 or 6 mm punch will usually be adequate. The punch is driven full thickness through the epithelial surface. The surrounding skin is pressed and the plug will pop outwards. This can be 'harpooned' with a fine needle (e.g. orange, No. 15). Taking care not to damage the overlying epithelium, the plug is lifted and snipped off at its base with scissors.
   b. *Surgical excision*—an elliptical excision is made with a 15 blade, preferably with the ellipse running along the circumference of the vulva, rather than radially. This is sewn up with soluble sutures such as 4/0 Vicryl. A protective sanitary towel should be supplied immediately post-operatively for any spotting. The vulva heals well with minimal scarring.

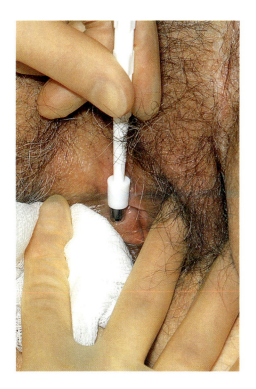

Figure 2.9

Punch biopsy. A 3 or 4 mm punch is driven full thickness through the epithelial surface.

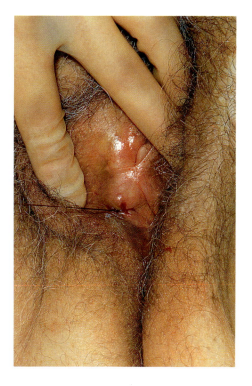

Figure 2.10

A soluble stitch may be necessary to achieve haemostasis.

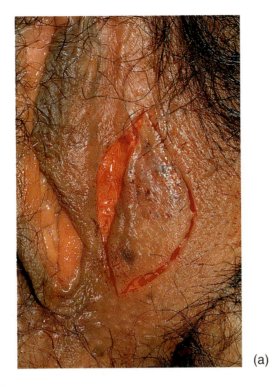

(a)

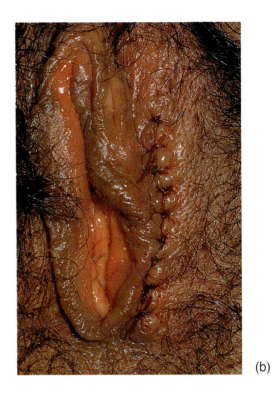

(b)

Figure 2.11

(a) Elliptical incision running around the
circumference of the vulva.

(b) The incision is sewn up with 4/0 Vicryl.

3 Commonly observed non-pathological lesions

There are a number of common non-pathological conditions that may be a source of distress to patients, but usually explanation and reassurance are all that is required.

Fordyce spots

Fordyce spots are simply normal yellowish sebaceous glands viewed through the labial

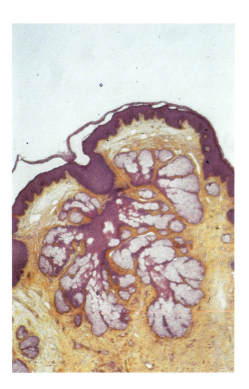

Figure 3.1
Histology of Fordyce spots. There is a proliferation of sebaceous glands opening directly on to the surface (H & E, ×40).

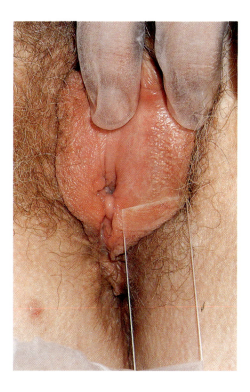

Figure 3.2
Fordyce spots on the inner aspect of the left labia minora.

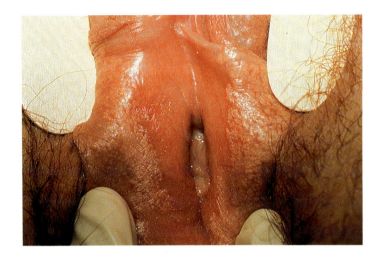

Figure 3.3
Fordyce spots. A florid example.

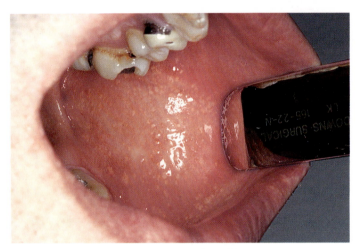

Figure 3.4
Fordyce spots. These may also be found in the mouth.

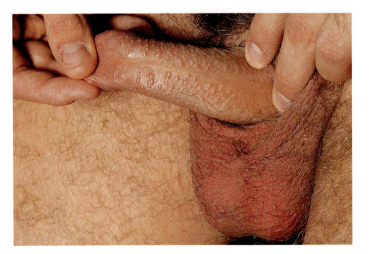

Figure 3.5
Fordyce spots on the shaft of the penis.

epithelium – the glands hypertrophy and hence become more easily visible at puberty and with pregnancy or hormonal treatment. Such glands can also be seen on the lips and oral mucosa. Patients often need reassurance that they are normal.

Angiokeratomata

Angiokeratomata are tiny clusters of dilated blood vessels surmounted by a peak of keratin. They can be bright red, but gradually darken to almost black with time. They are not seen until puberty, and thereafter last into old age. They are common, probably occurring in 1% of women. Similar lesions are seen on scrotal skin. They can easily be ablated by electrodesiccation or hyfrecation, half an hour after the application of local anaesthetic gel.

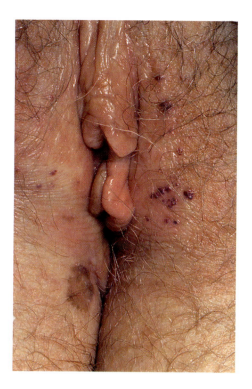

Figure 3.6

Angiokeratomata on the labia majora (note the seborrhoeic wart at 7 o'clock).

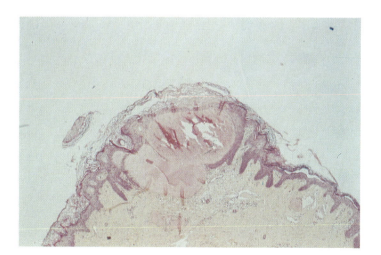

Figure 3.7

Histology of angiokeratoma. There are dilated capillaries in the papillary dermis stretching and effacing the overlying epidermis with surface hyperkeratosis (H & E, ×11).

Vulval papillomatosis

Vulval papillomatosis is a variant of normal. In some individuals the hormonal stimulation of puberty leads to unusually prominent thickening and folding of the labial epithelium. Such changes are very commonly seen in the second and third trimesters of pregnancy.

Vulval papillomatosis is often mistaken for human papilloma virus (HPV) infection. Extensive studies of many patients with histology and Southern blotting have failed to support evidence for any known HPV in the aetiology of this condition. Application of 4% acetic acid to such normal but hypertrophied epithelia can produce 'aceto-whitening'. This is not to be confused with aceto-whitening as seen in warts (warts are focal, asymmetrical and scattered). The biopsy can be similarly confusing to an inexperienced pathologist. The hypertrophied epithelium of the vestibule contains glycogen-rich pale cells which can be mistaken for the koilocytes seen in viral warts (see Figure 3.12).

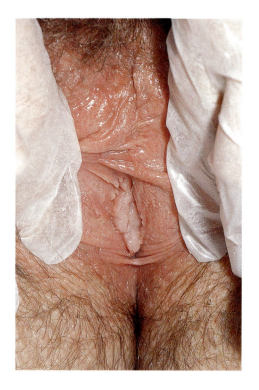

Figure 3.8
Vulval papillomatosis showing curious digitate lesions.

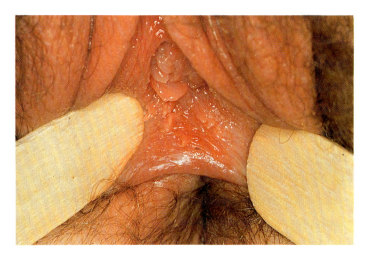

Figure 3.9
Vulval papillomatosis widely involving the vestibule and the labia minora.

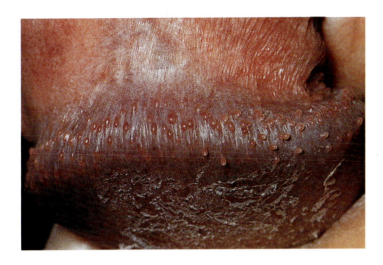

Figure 3.10

Penile Pearly Papules. This is the male equivalent of vulval papillomatosis. They are both harmless physiological variants of normal and require no treatment.

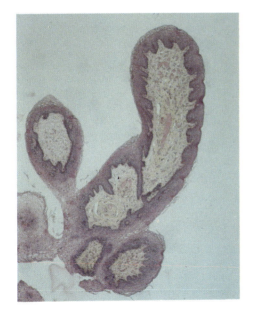

(a)

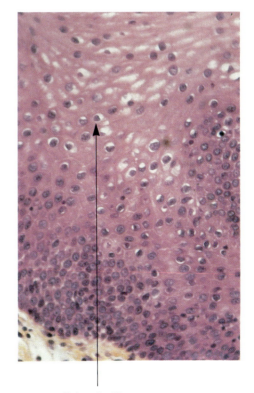

(b)

Figure 3.11

(a) Histology of finger-like papillomatosis (H & E, ×2). (b) Enlargement shows appearances which are often mistaken for koilocytosis; here the pallor is caused by glycogen-rich vestibular epithelial cells. Note the regularity of the nuclei (see Figure 3.12) (H & E, ×83).

Pale cell with regular and centrally placed nucleus.

Irregular nuclear
material eccentrically
placed.

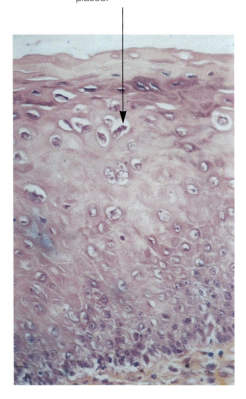

Figure 3.12

Koilocytosis, for comparison, demonstrates
irregular nuclear material eccentrically placed,
typical of papilloma virus infection (H & E, ×83).

4 Inflammatory diseases

This group of disorders constitutes the commonest diagnoses of those seeking consultation and thus the bulk of pathology seen in a vulval clinic. They are usually very symptomatic. Fortunately, correct diagnosis and treatment leads to dramatic improvement in most of these patients. (It should be noted that vulval skin, perhaps because of its flexural site, modifies the morphology of skin lesions somewhat, occasionally making prompt diagnosis difficult, even for experienced observers.)

Lichen sclerosus of the vulva

Lichen sclerosus is a destructive inflammatory condition with a predilection for genital skin. It occurs in both males and females and begins at any age. It can affect the whole genital skin (sometimes in a 'figure-of-eight' pattern), including the perianal area, and genitocrural folds. Interestingly, inflammation never extends to the vaginal mucosa.

The precise incidence of vulval lichen sclerosus is unknown. The provision of specialized vulval clinics has increased awareness, and a referral pattern has evolved showing that the disease is probably more common than was previously suspected.

There is a statistical association with other autoimmune conditions, particularly autoimmune thyroid disease. Rarely, extragenital skin involvement can occur.

The destructive inflammation usually causes pruritus intense enough to disturb sleep. However, a proportion of patients are asymptomatic. The condition is commonly misdiagnosed as recurrent candidiasis and the delay in diagnosis before referral to a vulval clinic is often many years. The physical signs, however, allow a definite and immediate clinical diagnosis to be made in most cases. The characteristic features are a whitening and scarring atrophy causing gradual destruction of normal vulval architecture; with burying of the clitoris, resorption of the labia minora and eventual narrowing of the introitus.

It was originally believed that the majority of prepubertal patients with lichen sclerosus went into remission at the time of puberty. However, this is now known not to be the case. More alarmingly, a proportion of children with lichen sclerosus are misdiagnosed as being the victims of child abuse. The physical signs of purpura, scarring and atrophy can understandably be misleading (see page 175).

A rare complication of lichen sclerosus is the development of squamous cell carcinoma. In clinical practice, the incidence is less than 4% of patients with lichen sclerosus. However, if pathological specimens of squamous carcinoma are examined, evidence of lichen sclerosus is found in over 60% of cases and must, therefore, be important in the aetiology of this malignancy.

Figures 4.8–4.28 show the progression of scarring and tissue resorption in progressive lichen sclerosus.

Management

1 The histology is confirmed by punch biopsy under local anaesthetic in the outpatient clinic (see Figures 2.9–2.11).

2 A carefully monitored very potent topical corticosteroid (Grade I—see Appendix III) is used nightly for 1–2 months, then intermittently (e.g. fortnightly) and then as required. Patients should be instructed that a small (30 g) tube should last 2–3 months.

3 A patient information leaflet is supplied and an explanation is given of the rationale of regular follow up at least annually (see Appendix IV).

4 The patient is told to use a soap substitute for washing (see Appendix II).

5 The patient is warned to re-attend if erosions persist or new 'warty' changes occur.

6 Asymptomatic cases should be treated and followed up in exactly the same way.

7 Surgery has no place in the management of uncomplicated disease.

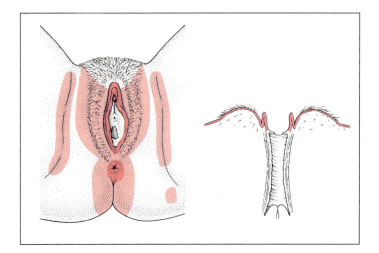

Figure 4.1

Distribution of lichen sclerosus. The darker sections denote the areas most commonly affected, the paler sections those less commonly affected.

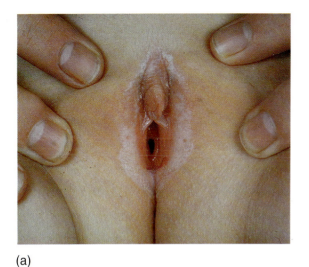

(a)

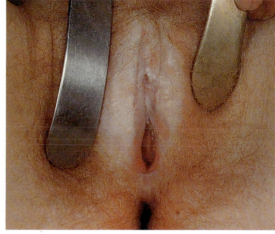

(b)

Figure 4.2

Lichen sclerosus. (a) Prepubertal vulval lichen sclerosus at the age of 7; note the well-demarcated whitening.

(b) The same patient, aged 20, shows progression of disease.

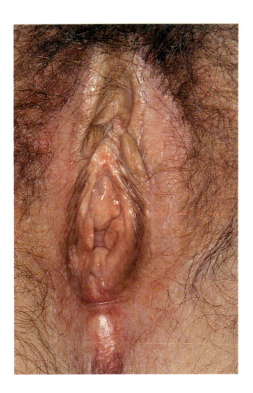

Figure 4.3

Lichen sclerosus. An early stage of disease showing resorption of the labia minora, but preservation of clitoral architecture.

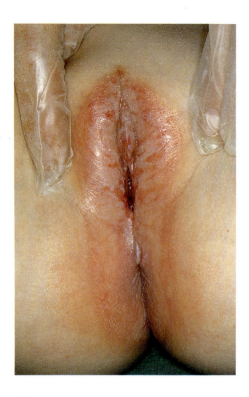

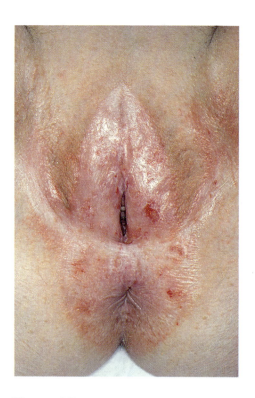

Figure 4.4

Lichen sclerosus in a 7-year-old, with extensive fissuring leading to painful micturition. Similarly, perianal involvement with fissuring often presents with constipation.

Figure 4.5

A postmenopausal patient with lichen sclerosus extending into perianal skin and genitocrural folds. The resorption of the labia minora can be seen.

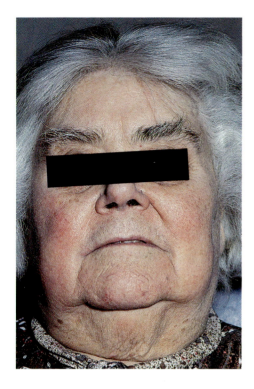

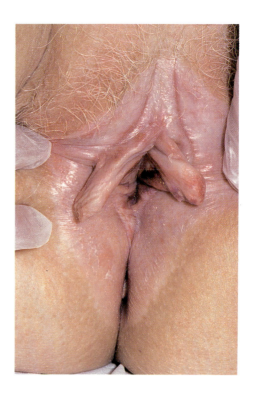

Figure 4.6

This patient with long-standing lichen sclerosus developed myxoedema, another auto-immune condition. Many patients have circulating auto-antibodies. Frank clinical disease is rare.

Figure 4.7

Typical lichen sclerosus with associated purpura.

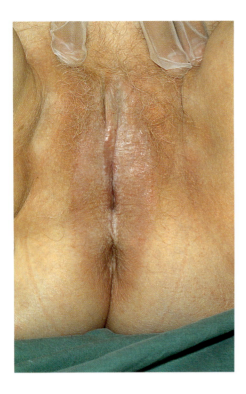

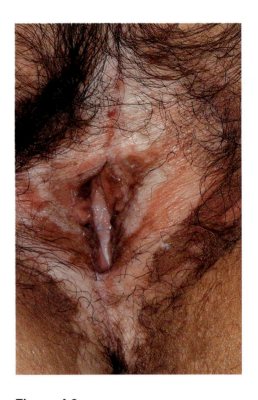

Figure 4.8

Advanced lichen sclerosus with loss of all normal architecture and the beginnings of introital narrowing. Note the glazed appearance of the atrophic skin.

Figure 4.9

Advanced lichen sclerosus, showing burying of clitoris and resorption of labia minora. Note the extensive loss of pigment and patchy post-inflammatory hyperpigmentation giving this variegated patterning.

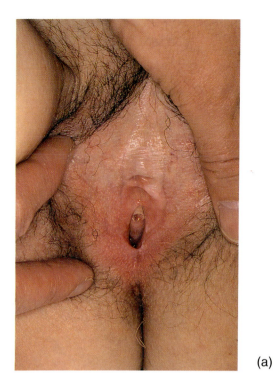

(a)

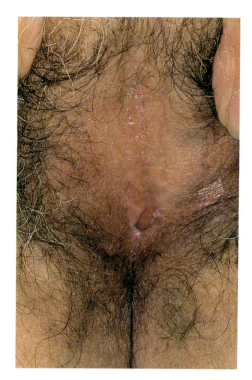

(b)

Figure 4.10

(a and b) Patient with lichen sclerosus showing progressive narrowing of the introitus, leaving only a tiny opening which leads to difficulties with micturition.

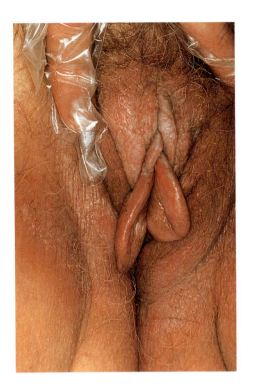

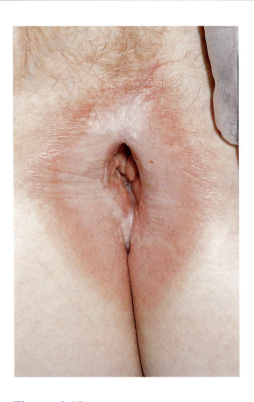

Figure 4.11

Lichen sclerosus may have an early erythematous phase and be mistaken for eczema. Biopsy, however, is helpful in this situation. This patient's biopsy showed the typical changes of lichen sclerosus (see Figure 4.23).

Figure 4.12

Vulvectomy was once considered to be a treatment option for lichen sclerosus. In the authors' experience, relapse following vulvectomy is the rule, as seen in this patient 5 years later.

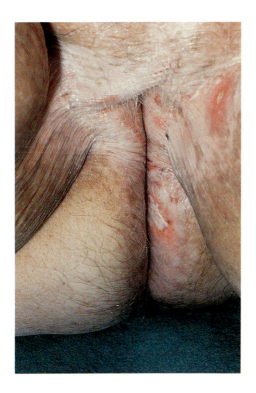

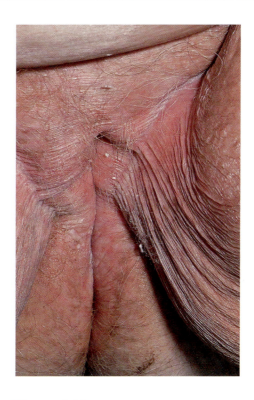

Figure 4.13

A 67-year-old woman with a 10-year history of severe pruritus vulvae despite Grade III/IV topical corticosteroids.

Figure 4.14

The same patient after 3 months of Grade I topical corticosteroid (clobetasol proprionate). Symptoms respond within days but adequate treatment helps prevent relapse (see page 20).

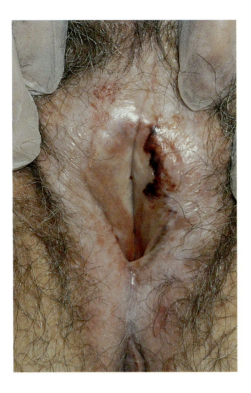

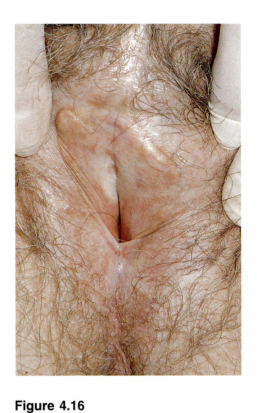

Figure 4.15

Lichen sclerosus with buried clitoris, resorbed labia and extensive purpura in a 53-year-old woman with a 15-year history of pruritus vulvae.

Figure 4.16

The same patient at 1-year follow-up. She had been treated with our standard regimen of nightly grade I topical corticosteroid for 2 months and had used less than 30 g over the year. Scarring is not reversed but symptoms are abolished and progression is halted.

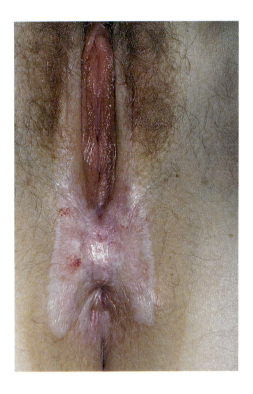

Figure 4.17
Lichen sclerosus is occasionally confined to the ridge of skin separating the vulva from the perianal area. Such patients often complain of dyspareunia, as they may tear at this site during sexual intercourse.

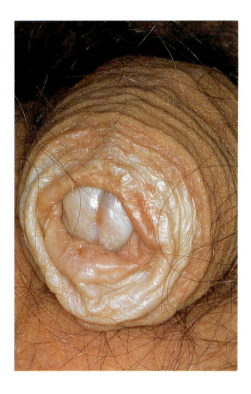

Figure 4.18
Lichen sclerosus affecting the male foreskin and glans. When scarring narrows the urethral orifice, the condition is referred to as balanitis xerotica obliterans.

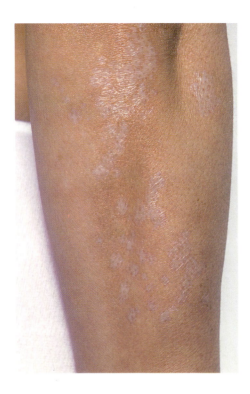

Figure 4.19

Extragenital lichen sclerosus. The typical 'white spot disease' appearance is seen. There is follicular delling, which is another helpful physical sign.

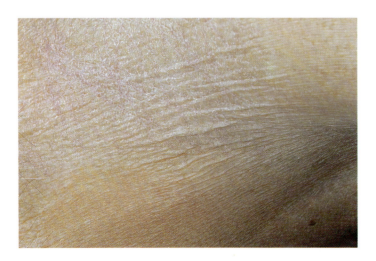

Figure 4.20

Extragenital lichen sclerosus with 'cigarette-paper' wrinkling.

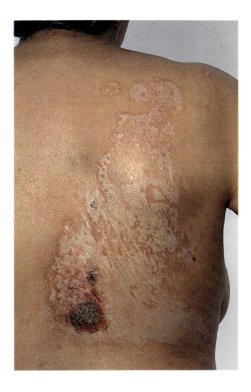

Figure 4.21
Extensive lichen sclerosus on the back, which is a common site for extra-genital disease. This patient had no involvement of genital skin. This is not unusual. Note also the purpura at an area where the dermo-epidermal junction has separated.

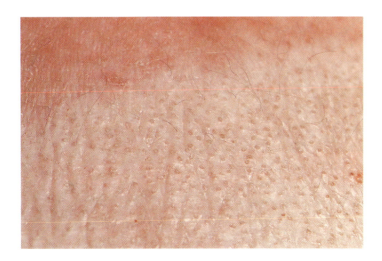

Figure 4.22
Close-up of extra-genital lichen sclerosus showing typical follicular delling and hyperkeratotic plugs.

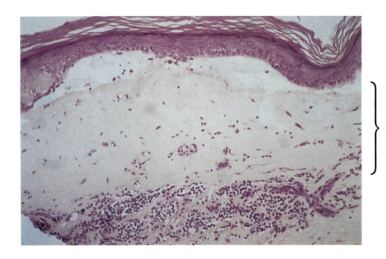

Superficial dermal hyalinization

Figure 4.23

Histology of lichen sclerosus. The classical features are
seen: an atrophic epidermis with an overlying
hyperkeratosis; an effaced dermo-epidermal junction;
superficial dermal hyalinization; and lymphocytic infiltrate
beneath the hyalinization (H & E, ×40).

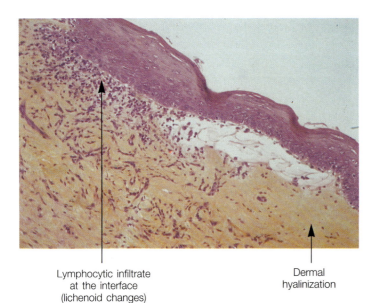

Lymphocytic infiltrate
at the interface
(lichenoid changes)

Dermal
hyalinization

Figure 4.24

Histology of lichen sclerosus. This
is an example of the lichenoid
changes that may be seen. A
lymphocytic infiltrate at the
interface, with basal cell
vacuolation and separation
(H & E, ×40).

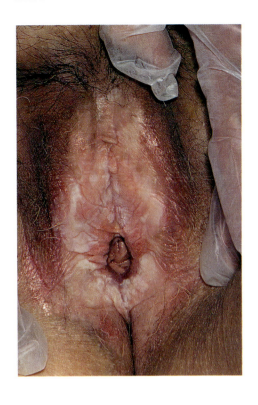

Figure 4.25

Lichen sclerosus complicated by an overlying benign hyperkeratotic epithelium. This is seen in about one-third of patients (see Figure 4.27).

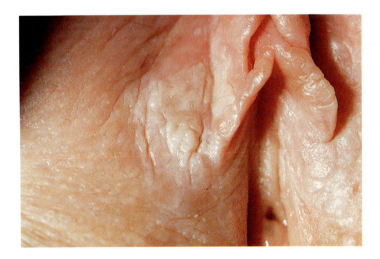

Figure 4.26

Closer view of a patient with benign hyperkeratosis overlying lichen sclerosus.

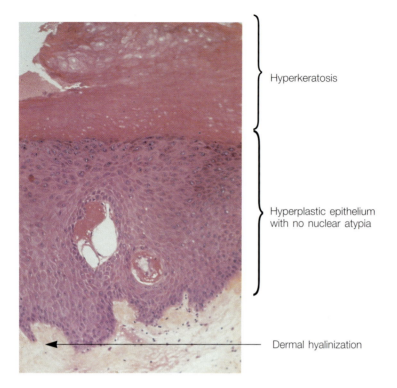

Hyperkeratosis

Hyperplastic epithelium
with no nuclear atypia

Dermal hyalinization

Figure 4.27
Histology of lichen sclerosus.
This is an example of lichen
sclerosus with an overlying
hyperplastic epithelium and
gross hyperkeratosis. Note
the underlying diagnostic
superficial dermal
hyalinization. This biopsy
came from the patient
illustrated in Figure 4.25

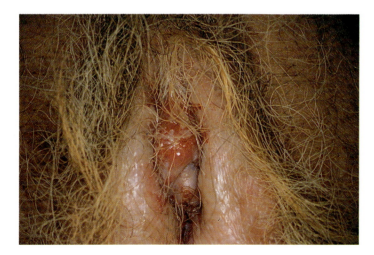

Figure 4.28
Lichen sclerosus complicated by
squamous cell carcinoma.

Seborrhoeic eczema

Seborrhoeic eczema is a common itchy, red, scaly eruption with a predilection for the face and scalp skin. A long history of intermittent scalp dandruff is usually obtained. Patients show poorly demarcated red patches in the seborrhoeic areas – the scalp, behind the ears, the sideboards and nasolabial folds. There is often marked scaling on an erythematous base to be seen in the eyebrows. The vulval itch is often out of proportion to the clinical signs found. Hence, it is worthwhile to check the scalp when the cause of pruritus vulvae is not immediately apparent.

A proportion of women with this common condition will have dermatitis on the body, particularly in occluded flexural areas, such as between the breasts, in the axillary vault and in vulval creases. Seborrhoeic eczema is a common cause of vulval pruritus where the dominant finding will be red, inflamed skin. The labia majora and surrounding perineal skin including the mons pubis are involved.

Itching leads to excoriations, lichenification and sometimes secondary infection.

Management

1   Swabs should be taken to exclude the possibility of secondary infection with either *Candida albicans* or pathogenic bacteria. The bacteria are best treated with systemic medications because topical antiseptics and antibiotics may cause sensitization.

2   A mild to moderate topical corticosteroid (Grades II or III—see Appendix III) will usually be effective, with improvement starting within a few days.

3   Lately, treatment aimed at reducing the level of commensal surface lipophilic yeasts (*Pityrosporum ovale*) has been advocated:

   a. *Topical treatment*
      i. Hairy areas—ketoconazole (e.g. Nizoral cream) or zinc pyrithione-containing shampoos.
      ii. Flexures—imidazole creams, sometimes in combination with topical corticosteroids: for example, 1% clotrimazole with 1% hydrocortisone (Canesten HC) or 2% miconazole nitrate with 1% hydrocortisone (Daktacort cream/Econacort ointment).

   b. *Systemic treatment*
      Tablets of fluconazole (e.g. 50 mg twice daily for 5 days), itraconazole (e.g. 100 mg twice daily for 5 days) or ketoconazole (e.g. 200 mg daily for a week) (nystatin, griseofulvin and terbinafine are not systemically active against *P. ovale*).

4   Most patients find a soap substitute helpful and should be advised to avoid irritants such as bubble-baths, shampoo in the bath and heavily fragranced soaps.

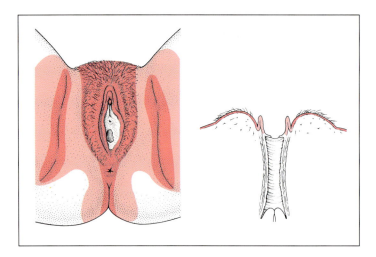

Figure 4.29
Distribution of seborrhoeic eczema.

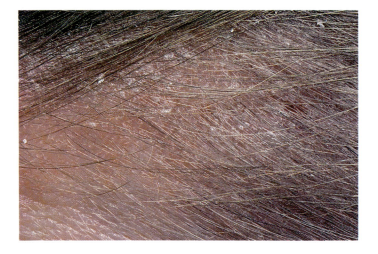

Figure 4.30
Seborrhoeic eczema. Examination
reveals diffuse fine scalp scaling.

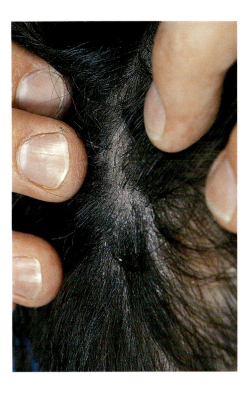

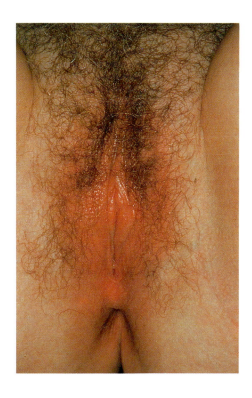

Figure 4.31
Seborrhoeic eczema. The scalp should always be examined when a patient presents with pruritus vulvae.

Figure 4.32
Seborrhoeic eczema. Note the poorly demarcated inflammation and lack of architectural disturbance in this mild example.

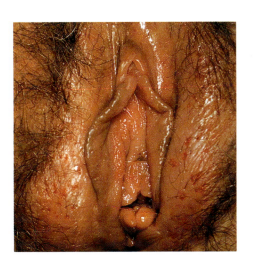

Figure 4.33
Seborrhoeic eczema. Scratching leads to excoriations.

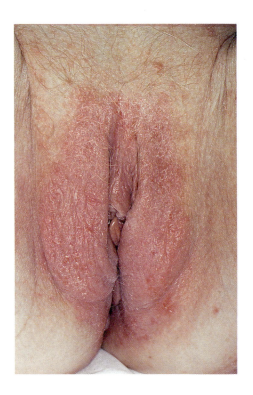

Figure 4.34

Seborrhoeic eczema. Long-term scratching has led to thickening of the skin of the labia majora (lichenification). This older patient has fewer hairs, and the erythema is more clearly seen.

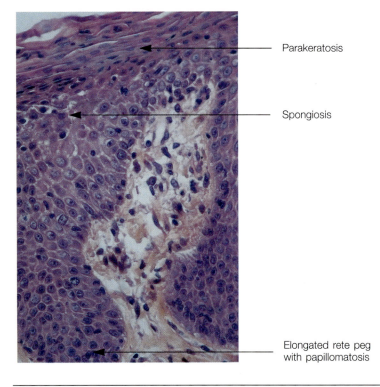

Parakeratosis

Spongiosis

Elongated rete peg
with papillomatosis

Figure 4.35

Histology of seborrhoeic eczema. The histology shows parakeratosis and papillomatosis reminiscent of psoriasis, but the absence of neutrophils infiltrating the epidermis and the presence of spongiosis and lymphocytic exocytosis help to confirm the diagnosis of seborrhoeic eczema (H & E, ×40).

Contact allergic eczema

The possibility of contact allergic eczema is often overlooked. Although uncommon, sensitization does occur and may be the cause of vulval itching and inflammation. Causative allergens include:

1 Medicaments (e.g. neomycin, ethylene diamine, local anaesthetics and cortico-steroids)
2 Rubber (e.g. condoms)
3 Other chemicals (e.g. spermicides and perfumes).
4 Nail varnish (there is seldom any reaction to be seen on the fingers themselves, but eyelids and neck may show eczematous patches).

Management

1 Patch testing facilities are available at most dermatology clinics and should be performed if contact sensitivity is suspected. All of the patient's topical preparations, as well as the Standard European Battery of Allergens, should be tested.
2 The culprit allergen is removed and avoided.
3 Grade II or, in severe cases, Grade I topical corticosteroids (see Appendix III) are prescribed.
4 In very severe cases, a 5-day course of systemic steroids, e.g. prednisolone 30 mg/day and gradually reducing.
5 In acute weeping eczema, potassium permanganate soaks are useful (see Appendix II).

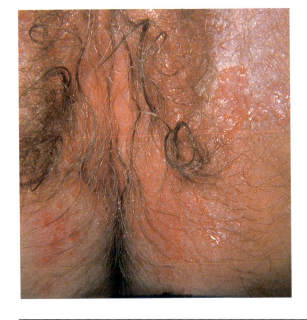

Figure 4.36
Acute contact allergic eczema. This case was due to allergy to a local anaesthetic (benzocaine).

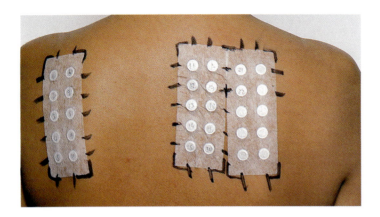

Figure 4.37
Patch tests are applied to a patient's back and removed to be read 48 hours later.

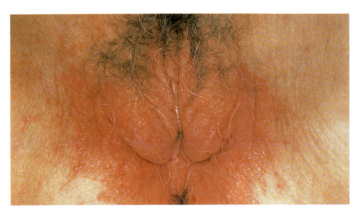

Figure 4.38
Contact allergic eczema. This patient's seborrhoeic eczema failed to respond to medication and patch testing revealed her to be allergic to the ethylenediamine present in her prescribed cream.

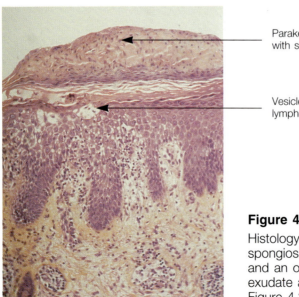

Parakeratotic scale with serous exudate

Vesicle containing lymphocytes

Figure 4.39
Histology of contact allergic eczema. Epidermal spongiosis and vesiculation, lymphocytic exocytosis and an overlying parakeratotic scale and serous exudate are seen in this histology from the patient in Figure 4.38 (H & E, ×40).

Irritant eczema

Eczema and inflammation can be caused by primary irritants. Worry over possible sexually acquired disease or attempts to minimize personal odour can lead to overenthusiastic cleansing with soaps and other products, with consequent damage to the epithelium. There is usually accompanying involvement of the genitocrural folds, as shown in Figure 4.40.

Management

1 Rinsing and removal of all traces of the irritant chemical if necessary.
2 Grade I topical corticosteroids (see Appendix III) can be used for up to a week.
3 Potassium permanganate soaks are useful (see Appendix II).

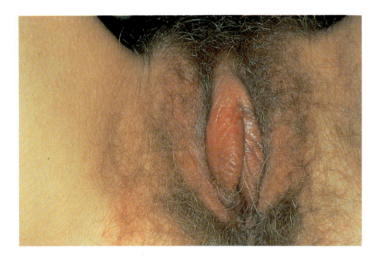

Figure 4.40

Irritant eczema. Caustic burn of the vulva caused by quaternary ammonium disinfectant (available as powders and solutions).

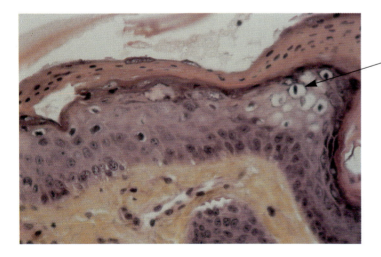

Vacuolation of the epidermal cells with no spongiosis, and no exocytosis

Figure 4.41

Histology of irritant eczema. This example, taken from the patient in Figure 4.40, shows vacuolation of the epidermal cells with overlying parakeratosis and no exocytosis (H & E, ×83).

Lichen simplex chronicus

Lichen simplex chronicus or neurodermatitis, is a very common cause of vulval symptomatology. Chronic rubbing and friction lead to thickening of the epithelium (histologically acanthosis). Most often, such 'habit scratching' leads to a visible area of thickened red skin. This is often asymmetrical and most commonly occurs in an area accessible to the dominant hand.

Management

1   Reassurance and explanation are the foundation of management. A confrontational approach to this 'self-induced' disease is seldom helpful.
2   Short-term Grades I or II topical corticosteroids (see Appendix III) may help to break the habit of scratching.
3   Patients should understand that their 'itch–scratch' cycle may recur at times of stress.

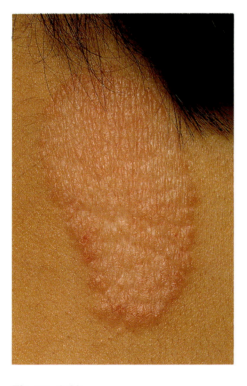

Figure 4.42
Lichen simplex chronicus on an accessible site at right side of back of neck.

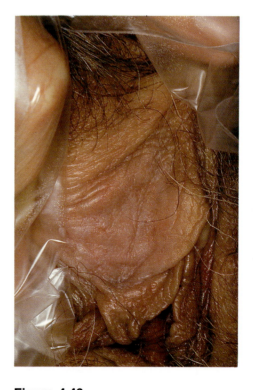

Figure 4.43
Lichen simplex chronicus. Well-demarcated patch of lichenification on the right interlabial sulcus.

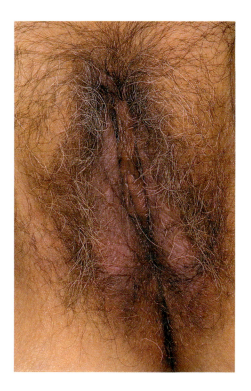

Figure 4.44

More extensive lichen simplex chronicus. Patients may deny scratching.

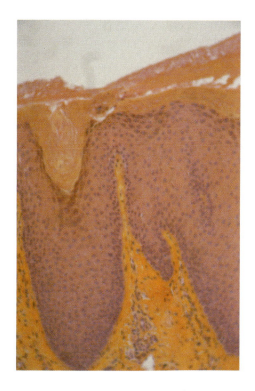

Figure 4.45

Histology of lichen simplex chronicus. There is marked thickening of the epidermis (acanthosis) with epidermal ridges projecting deep down into the dermis with rounded, burgeoning tips. No nuclear atypia is seen. There are occasional patches of spongiosis and overlying parakeratosis (H & E, ×40).

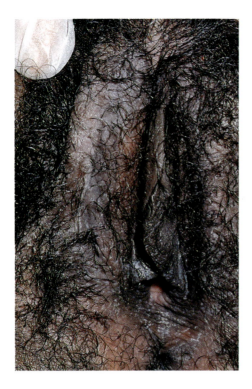

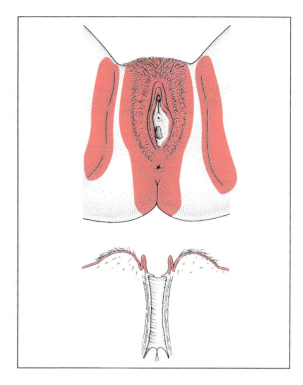

Figure 4.46
Lichen simplex. The thickened plaque visible on the right labia majora is bluish-pale in this black woman with a 2-year history of severe vulval itch.

Figure 4.47
Distribution of psoriasis.

Psoriasis

Psoriasis is notoriously chronic, and patients understandably fear this diagnosis. Lesions in the perineum are common and may cause difficulty in diagnosis, because in this occluded flexural site the familiar silver-scaled plaque appears as an inflamed 'beefy-red' area. Close inspection shows the characteristic uniform, symmetrical appearance and well-defined edge.

Any part of the perineum can be affected, but never the vaginal mucosa.

Support for the diagnosis should be sought in the elbows, knees, sacrum and scalp. The nails should be checked for signs of psoriasis – thimble pitting, subungual hyperkeratosis and onycholysis. However, anogenital lesions may be the only manifestations of the patient's psoriasis.

Psoriasis is common—there is a genetic predisposition in some 5% of the population, expressed clinically by some 2% at any one time. Precipitating factors include recent streptococcal infection (usually guttate psoriasis), and lesions may appear at sites of trauma (the Koebner phenomenon).

A characteristic psoriasis-like eruption is seen in Reiter's syndrome (see page 118).

Management

1 Full explanation and reassurance about the non-infectious nature of psoriasis is essential.

2 The patient should be educated that scratching exacerbates and perpetuates psoriatic plaques.

3 Irritation can occur, particularly in the deep folds of flexural psoriasis and the use of a soap substitute is thus often helpful, sometimes with the addition of coal tar solution (e.g. 10% coal tar solution in emulsifying ointment applied before bathing). Swabs should be taken as indicated to exclude secondary candidiasis.

4 Topical corticosteroids, although not generally recommended for extensive plaque psoriasis elsewhere on the skin, are particularly useful in flexural areas. A moderately potent corticosteroid with or without the addition of coal tar solution is often employed.

5 Dithranol and calcipotriol both have a narrow irritant/therapeutic ratio. Irritation is potentiated at sites of natural occlusion, therefore these preparations should be avoided in the anogenital region. The newer vitamin D analogue, tacalcitol, is less irritant and helps considerably in a proportion of patients.

6 Patients with severe and extensive psoriasis may require second-line treatments (e.g. weekly oral methotrexate, oral retinoids or cyclosporin A). Flexural sites can be confidently expected to respond equally well. These patients should be under the supervision of a specialist for such prescriptions to be considered.

7 Some drugs exacerbate psoriasis, for example lithium succinate, chloroquine and beta-blockers.

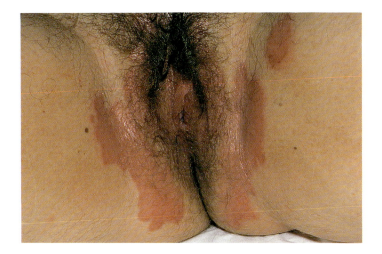

Figure 4.48
Psoriasis affecting the labia and extending into the genitocrural folds.

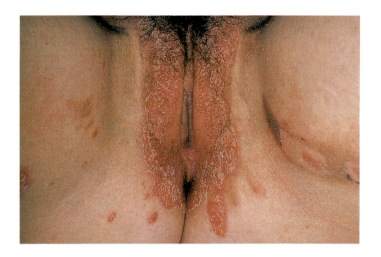

Figure 4.49
Psoriasis of the labia majora. Note
the crisp demarcation and, in this
case, scaling. There are also
typical plaques of psoriasis
scattered on the inner thighs.

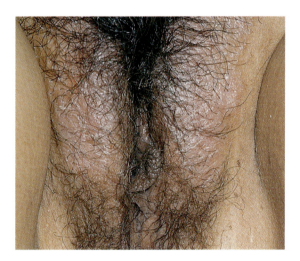

Figure 4.50
Psoriasis on the labia majora of a 24-year-old
Asian woman.

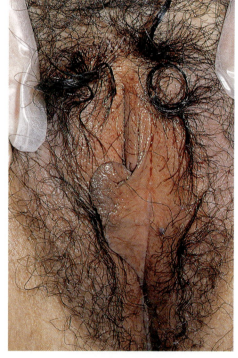

Figure 4.51
The same patient 2 months later, showing an
excellent response to topical tacalcitol.

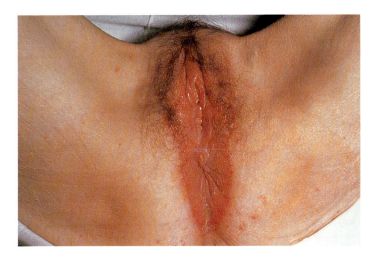

Figure 4.52

Flexural psoriasis showing glistening moist inflammation. The well-demarcated edge helps in diagnosis; lesions can be seen extending into the perianal skin.

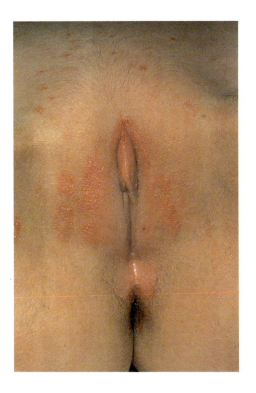

Figure 4.53

Psoriasis, confined to the vulva, presenting for the first time at puberty.

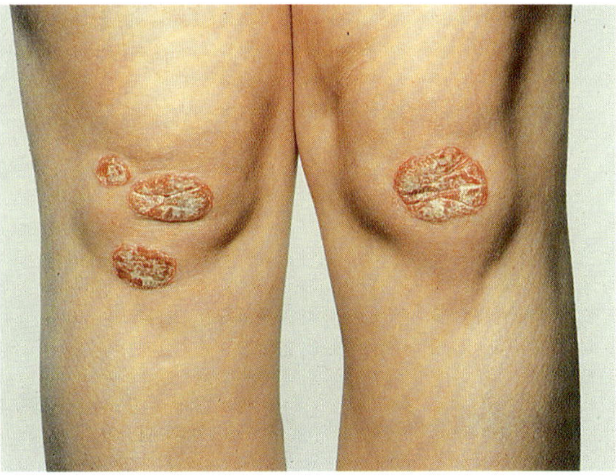

Figure 4.54

Typical psoriasis of knees.

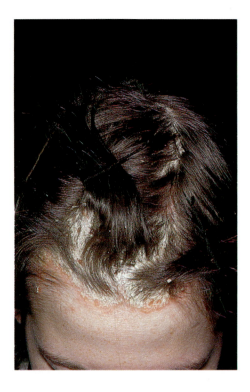

Figure 4.55

Typical psoriasis of the scalp. The diagnosis of psoriasis is aided by checking the characteristic sites of knees, elbows, sacrum and scalp.

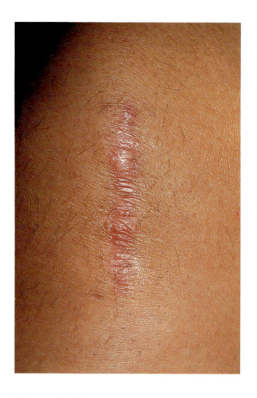

Figure 4.56

Koebner phenomenon. Psoriasis often emerges in areas of damaged skin, here in a surgical wound.

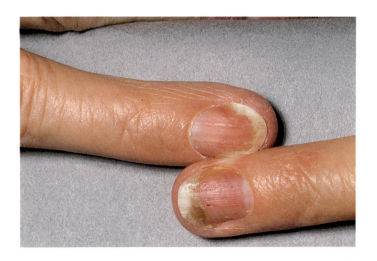

Figure 4.57

Evidence of psoriasis in the nails, with thimble pitting, onycholysis and dystrophy, should be sought.

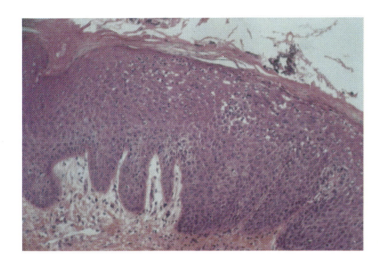

(a)

Figure 4.58

Histology of vulval psoriasis.
(a) There is papillomatosis, parakeratosis, neutrophil exocytosis and spongiform pustules (H & E, ×40).
(b) Enlargement shows neutrophil exocytosis and spongiform pustules in more detail (H & E, ×83).

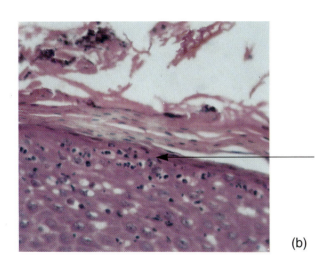

(b)

Neutrophil exocytosis and spongiform pustules

Lichen planus (papular variety)

Cutaneous papular lichen planus is an inflammatory skin condition causing intensely pruritic violaceous shiny papules distributed widely on the skin. Similar papules can occur on the vulval skin. Papules occur on the labia majora and genitocrural folds. The vestibule and vagina are spared. Mucosal lesions are common in the mouth, but rare in the genital tract.

The aetiology is unknown but thought to involve lymphocyte-mediated autoimmune destruction of the epithelial basal cells. Lichen planus is seen in some patients with other autoimmune conditions such as primary biliary cirrhosis. Similar histopathology and clinical lesions can be seen as part of chronic graft-versus-host disease following bone marrow transplantation.

Lichen planus is rare in childhood and old age and usually affects 25–40 year olds. Untreated papular lesions gradually resolve leaving pigmented tattoos over 12–24 months. Occasionally scarring occurs. Renewed cropping in later years may occur.

Erosive lichen planus, a very rare condition, is discussed in the next section.

Management

1 The histology is confirmed by punch biopsy (see Figures 2.9–2.11).
2 Grade I topical corticosteroids should be applied nightly (see Appendix III). The patient is reviewed every 3 weeks until symptoms are relieved and the raised papular elements have flattened. Treatment should *not* be continued for pigmentary changes.
3 Reassurance of the benign non-infectious nature of the condition, and a full explanation of the tendency for natural resolution after 6–18 months, is important. It should be explained that the condition may heal, leaving marked pigmentary changes that may take many years to resolve.
4 A patient information leaflet should be supplied (see Appendix IV).

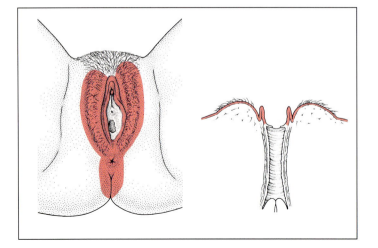

Figure 4.59
Distribution of cutaneous papular lichen planus.

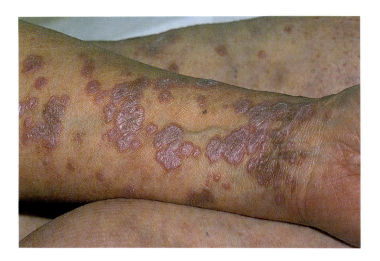

Figure 4.60

Lichen planus showing typical flat-topped violaceous papules, affecting the volar aspect of the wrist of this patient. Other characteristic sites include scalp, sacrum, axillae, mouth and nails.

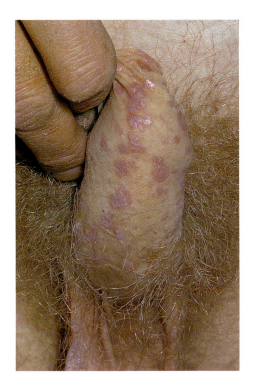

Figure 4.61

Lichen planus. Lesions similar to those in Figure 4.60, on the shaft of the penis.

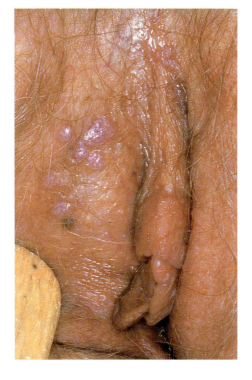

Figure 4.62

Typical papular lichen planus affecting the labia majora. Note the violaceous colour and white Wickham's striae.

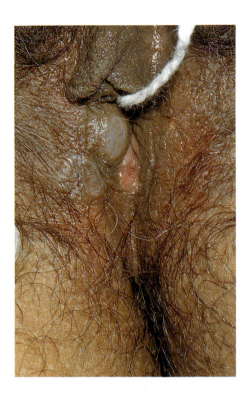

Figure 4.63
Lichen planus. An Arabian woman with two areas of
cutaneous papular lichen planus. Note the upper lesion
spreading onto the vestibular surface; the lower lesion
has a typical annular configuration. Histology was
characteristic.

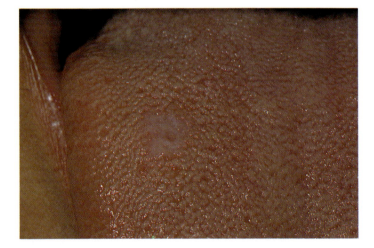

Figure 4.64
Lichen planus lesion on the tongue
(same patient as in Figure 4.63).

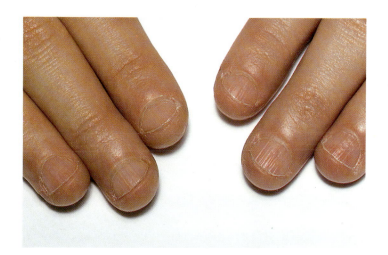

Figure 4.65

Lichen planus nail dystrophy. Nails showing longitudinal ridging.

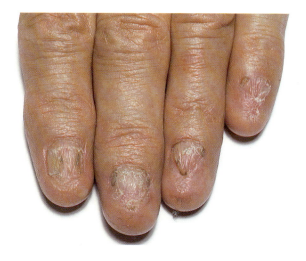

Figure 4.66

Lichen planus nail dystrophy. A more advanced case showing scarring, with pterygium deformity.

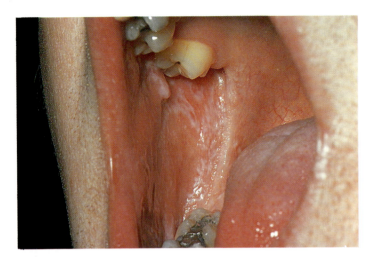

Figure 4.67

Mucosal lichen planus. Mouth of a patient with lichen planus, showing the lace-like white streaks seen in the non-erosive phase.

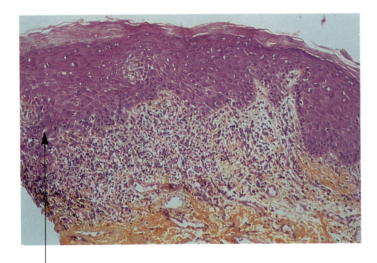

Basal cell
liquefaction

Figure 4.68

Histology of lichen planus. There is basal cell liquefaction at the dermo-epidermal junction with a heavy band-like subepidermal lymphocytic infiltrate (H & E, ×40).

Erosive vulvo-vagino-gingival lichen planus (Syndrome of Hewitt and Pelisse)

Erosive vulvo-vagino-gingival lichen planus (Syndrome of Hewitt and Pelisse) is a rare condition. It presents with painful mucosal erosions which rapidly lead to scarring. Erosions are confined to the vestibule and vagina and are rarely associated with cutaneous disease even when the mouth and gingivae are severely affected.

Erosive lichen planus is much more resistant to treatment with steroids than is lichen sclerosus, and it is best managed in specialized vulval clinics.

Management

1 The diagnosis is confirmed by punch biopsy (see Figures 2.9–2.11). Biopsies must be taken from the edge of the lesions rather than from erosions, to obtain diagnostic changes.

2 Swabs are taken to exclude secondary infection and appropriate treatment given if necessary.

3 Reassurance of the non-infectious nature of the condition and explanation should be given.

4 Antiseptic soaks such as diluted potassium permanganate may be soothing and helpful (see Appendix II).

5 The first-line treatment for erosive disease is potent topical corticosteroids. Erosions which fail to respond or become deeply ulcerated should be subjected to biopsy to exclude invasive neoplastic change.

   a. *Vaginal erosions*—topical corticosteroids designed for vaginal use are not available. However, some of the preparations used for the treatment of proctitis or ulcerative colitis may be used, for example suppository and foam steroid preparations.

   b. *Vulval erosions*—Grade I topical corticosteroids are used. Some preparations may be poorly tolerated. Creams spread on to alginate dressings applied to eroded surfaces and changed regularly may be more satisfactory.

6 Systemic steroids are not often helpful, and correctly applied and carefully monitored Grade I topical corticosteroids are usually more successful.

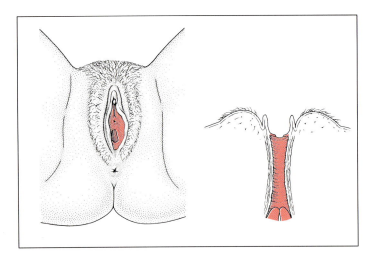

Figure 4.69
Distribution of erosive lichen planus.

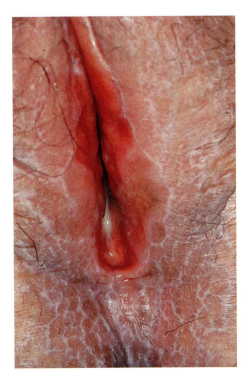

Figure 4.70
Erosive lichen planus of the vestibule showing loss of labia minora and Wickham's striae extending out into the perineal skin.

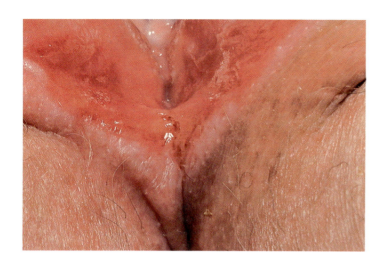

Figure 4.71
Erosive lichen planus of the vulva and vagina showing synechiae formation, which is not uncommon in this condition.

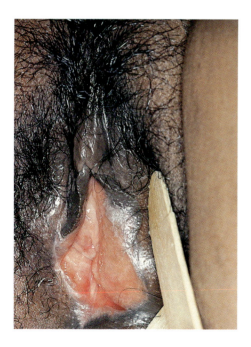

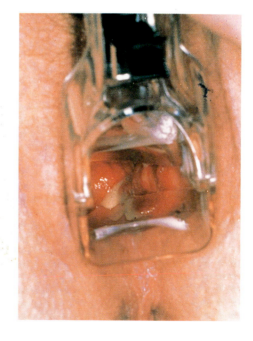

Figure 4.72
Erosive lichen planus – a distressingly painful condition, often poorly responsive to treatment.

Figure 4.73
Erosive lichen planus. Speculum examination of the vagina is often impossible, but will reveal an erythematous friable and eroded epithelium. Scarring can lead to vaginal stenosis.

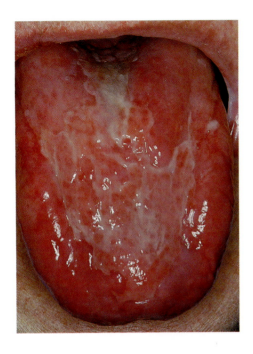

Figure 4.74
Erosive lichen planus affecting the tongue.

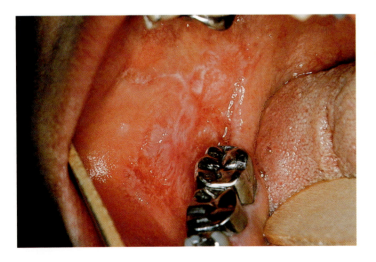

Figure 4.75
Erosive lichen planus affecting the inner cheek; note the background lace-like pattern.

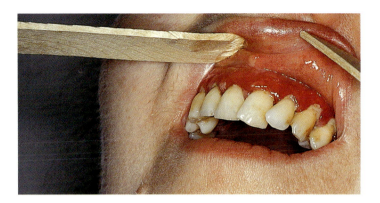

Figure 4.76
Erosive lichen planus of the gums,
which may be asymptomatic.

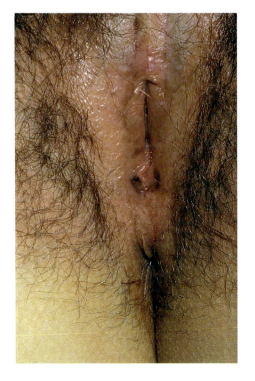

Figure 4.77
Post-inflammatory hyperpigmentation, a common
sequelae of healed erosive lichen planus.

Vacuolation of the
majority of basal
cells with incipient
blister formation

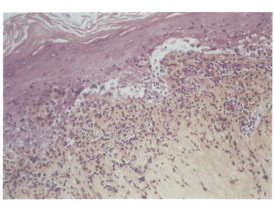

(a)

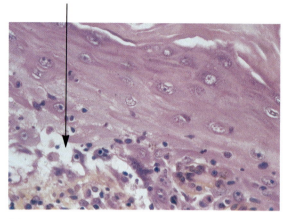

(b)

Figure 4.78

Histology of erosive lichen planus. (a) This
example shows a dense lymphocytic infiltrate
effacing the dermo-epidermal junction with a
thin, flattened epithelium. There is vacuolation
of all basal cells and incipient blister formation
(H & E, ×40). (b) Enlargement of the same
specimen (H & E, ×83).

Vestibulitis

Vestibulitis was first recognized in the late nineteenth century, and then disappeared from the literature until recently. Interestingly, patients are often fair-skinned redheads with a history of sensitive skin at other sites, commonly the face. This condition is characterized by a triad of dyspareunia, vulval vestibular erythema and tenderness to palpation. Its aetiology is unknown and it is not due to inflammation of the minor vestibular gland, as was once thought. The patient may also complain of urinary symptoms such as dysuria and strangury. The pain is precipitated by intercourse or the insertion of a tampon. On examination there may be erythema, confined to areas lateral to the hymenal ring or over the introitus. If the areas are touched with a cotton bud, pain will be induced and the erythema will intensify or appear for the first time. Occasionally numerous papillae may be seen (vestibular papillomatosis – see discussion on page 16), which are commonly misinterpreted as vulval warts (see Figure 3.12). These papillae are confined to the inner aspects of the labia minora and vestibule; they can arise from a solitary base, but, unlike warts, they do not coalesce. Their distribution is even and symmetrical. Studies of papillomatosis have failed to show evidence of known human papilloma virus types, and it is thought to be an anatomical variant in normal patients. Its presence in cases of vestibulitis is therefore coincidental.

Management

1 Patients are reassured to learn that vestibulitis is a recognizable condition, and that it is not a primary psychological problem. There is really no satisfactory treatment, and the usual recommendation is to use a soap substitute and to avoid soaps and bubble baths. The majority of patients do well, and with time their symptoms lessen and eventually resolve. Those that do not and have incapacitating symptoms should be carefully assessed for underlying psychological problems.

2 There is frequently an intolerance to topical medications, but patch testing is invariably negative. Specific treatment with oral imidazoles, metronidazole and tetracyclines is unhelpful.

3 5% Lignocaine ointment can prove of temporary benefit, and in some patients an antihistamine may also help.

4 A tricyclic antidepressant can be used mainly for its central effect on pain, but also for its effect on secondary depression.

5 Surgical ablation of the vestibular gland-bearing area, by either excision or laser, has been reported to lead to an improvement in selected patients, but there are no good long-term follow-up studies.

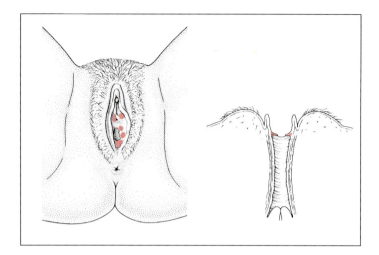

Figure 4.79
Distribution of vestibulitis.

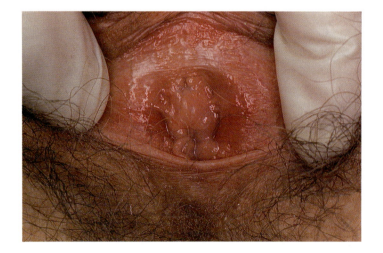

Figure 4.80
Vestibulitis. Erythema is localized to the vestibule at the site of the openings of Bartholin's glands (5 and 7 o'clock). The erythematous areas can be tested for tenderness with a cotton bud.

5 Ulcerating and blistering disorders

This group of disorders usually causes pain rather than itch, and is much rarer than the inflammatory diseases discussed in the preceding chapter. It is very important to examine other mucous membranes for evidence of disease. Biopsy with specialized immunofluorescent pathology is usually required to establish the diagnosis, and often the advice of specialist colleagues (e.g. ophthalmic and oral medicine surgeons) may be required with diagnosis and management.

Aphthae

Aphthous ulcers of the mouth are a common phenomenon in healthy young adults. Genital involvement is less common, but does occur.

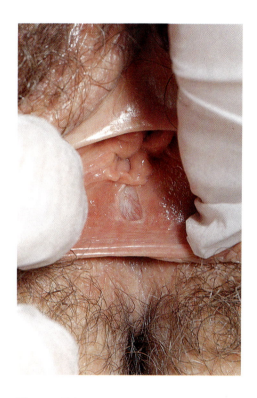

Figure 5.1
Acutely painful aphthous ulcer presenting with dyspareunia. Virology and bacteriology were negative. Treatment was conservative.

Management

1   Soothing antiseptic soaks with diluted potassium permanganate are helpful (see Appendix II).
2   Grade I topical corticosteroids are often helpful (see Appendix III).
3   Steroid injections intralesionally just beneath the ulcer base may help, e.g. triamcinolone acetonide 10 mg/ml (Adcortyl).
4   Courses of minocycline can be tried. This gives benefit in a proportion of patients (presumably due to its anti-inflammatory properties).

Lesions can attain quite a large size. Swabs should always be taken to exclude herpes simplex. Patients of a certain HLA type may be more prone to aphthae, but the cause of these aphthae remains unknown.

Behçet's disease

Behçet's disease is a rare condition, more common in the Near East, characterized by deep painful mucosal ulcers ('giant aphthae'). Deep ulceration of the genitalia may be accompanied by fever, prostration, pathergy and crops of follicular lesions. Rarely, ocular and neurological lesions occur.

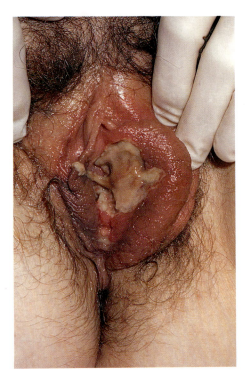

Figure 5.2
Behçet's disease. Extensive deep ulcers penetrating the labia.

Management

1   Diagnosis is by exclusion of other possible diseases, especially infections. Swabs are mandatory.
2   Biopsy will only show non-specific ulceration and secondary changes.
3   Soothing antiseptic soaks, such as diluted potassium permanagate solution are helpful (see Appendix II).
4   When the lesions are eroded, Grade I topical corticosteroids (see Appendix III) are sometimes better tolerated when applied as a layer on alginate dressings, or when mixed: e.g. Dermovate (clobetasol propionate) ointment mixed equal parts with Orabase. Steroid injections intralesionally just beneath the ulcer base may help, e.g. triamcinolone acetonide 10 mg/ml (Adcortyl).
5   Oral thalidomide can be dramatically beneficial, but the risk of teratogenicity and nerve damage must always be borne in mind. Availability of this drug is very limited, but it can usually be obtained for special circumstances.
6   Severe disease, especially ocular disease, is usually treated with systemic steroids.

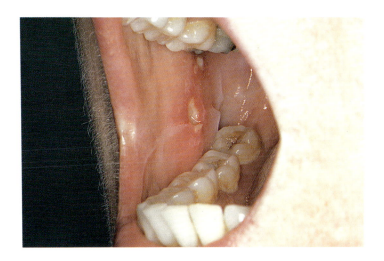

Figure 5.3
Behçet's disease. Deep mouth ulcers in the same patient as in Figure 5.2.

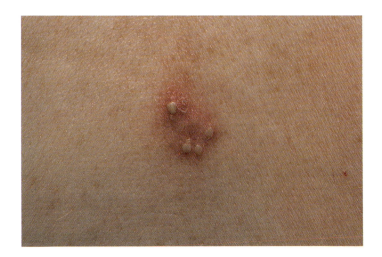

Figure 5.4
Behçet's disease. Groups of pustular folliculitis may be found on the trunk, as shown here on the back of the same patient as in Figures 5.2 and 5.3.

Erythema multiforme

Erythema multiforme is an acute skin reaction pattern, usually lasting approximately a fortnight. In mild cases, small round areas of erythema on the extremities are accompanied by painful mucosal lesions. In severe cases, extensive bullous lesions, sometimes leading to chronic scarring, can occur (the Stevens–Johnson syndrome). Erythema multiforme can occur 8–10 days after antigenic stimulation, such as a viral infection with herpes simplex or drug exposure; but in approximately half the patients, no cause is found.

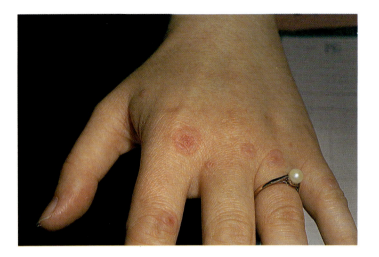

Figure 5.5
Erythema multiforme. Typical target lesions affecting the dorsum of the hand.

Management

1   The triggering event is addressed; for example drug avoidance, suppression of recurrent herpes simplex virus with long-term acyclovir, etc.
2   Oral or ocular involvement should be carefully evaluated and treated.
3   Grade I topical corticosteroid (see Appendix III) can be used for 1–2 weeks.
4   Short courses of systemic steroids reduce fever, toxicity and ease local pain, e.g. prednisolone 40 mg/day reducing over 6 days.
5   Local cooling antiseptic soaks, such as diluted potassium permanganate, are helpful (see Appendix II).

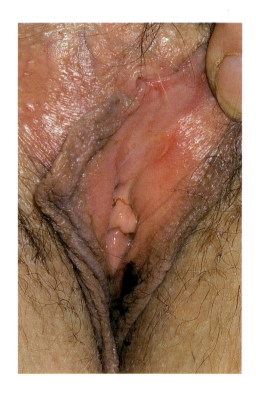

Figure 5.6
Erythema multiforme. Target lesions similar to those in Figure 5.5 (and in the same patient) causing an erosion on the inner aspect of the labia minora.

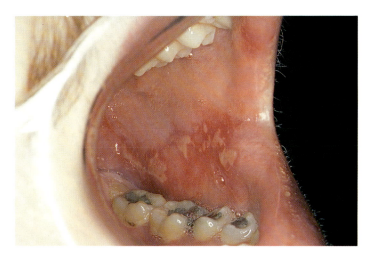

Figure 5.7

Extensive oral involvement in erythema multiforme. This woman's erythema multiforme occurred 8 days after ingestion of a non-steroidal anti-inflammatory agent.

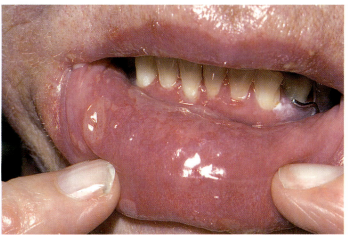

Figure 5.8

Typical bullous erythema multiforme lesions in the mouth. In this case, the lesions were triggered by sulphonamide.

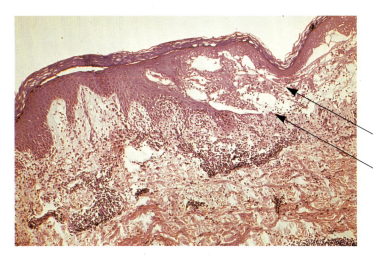

Figure 5.9

Histology of erythema multiforme. There is severe epidermal necrosis with subepidermal fibrin exudation and heavy dermal lymphocytic infiltration (H & E, ×40).

Necrotic epidermis

Blister filled with fibrin and lymphocytes

Toxic epidermal necrolysis (Lyell's syndrome)

Toxic epidermal necrolysis (TEN) is an even more severe form of superficial reactive infarction which may cause extensive blistering and erosion of the skin and mucosal surfaces. Hypersensitivity to drugs is the usual cause, for example non-steroidal anti-inflammatory agents, carbamazepine, phenytoin, co-trimoxazole, dapsone and sulpha drugs. A less severe and more superficial variant is seen in childhood which is caused by staphylococcal exotoxin—the staphylococcal scalded skin syndrome.

Management

1 General
   a. The cause is identified and removed.
   b. Early transfer of patients to a high-dependency treatment unit, before severe generalized blistering occurs, is essential.
   c. The use of systemic steroids in very severe generalized toxic epidermal necrolysis is controversial, as there is evidence to suggest that their use leads to increased mortality due to serious infections.
   d There are anecdotal reports of the successful use of cyclosporin-A.
2 Vulval lesions
   a. Local soothing and antiseptic soaks are applied to the vulva, for example diluted potassium permanganate (see Appendix II).
   b. Topical Grade I corticosteroids are prescribed and carefully monitored (see Appendix III).

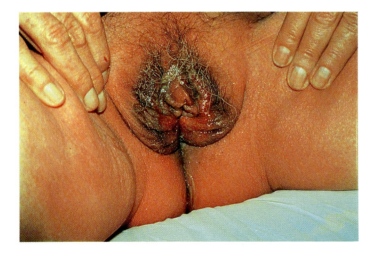

Figure 5.10
Vulval TEN showing severe erosion and necrosis in a patient taking a non-steroidal anti-inflammatory drug.

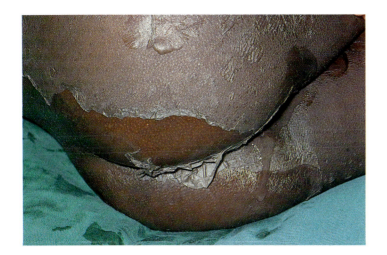

Figure 5.11
Vulval TEN showing severe
blistering, exudation and
widespread peeling.

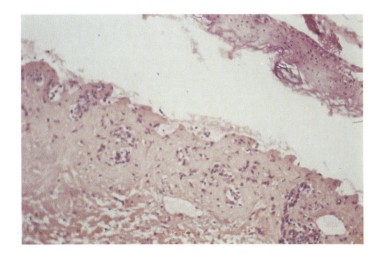

Figure 5.12
Histology of TEN. There is necrosis
of the epidermis, subepidermal
blistering with relatively sparse
lymphocytic inflammatory infiltration
(H & E, ×40).

Fixed drug eruption

In this condition, asymmetrical patches of intense inflammation occur both on skin and mucosal surfaces each time the offending drug is taken. Patients rarely associate the eruption with the ingestion of the agent, which may be a proprietary substance, for example phenolphthalein in a laxative or codeine in an analgesic. The vulval mucosa is commonly affected. Other drugs imputed include paracetamol, nonsteroidal anti-inflammatory agents, tetracycline, griseofulvin and cytotoxic agents. A challenge results in reaction at exactly the same sites within 24 hours. Healing leaves darkly pigmented patches which remain as evidence for months.

Management

1   Avoidance of the triggering drug is curative (hypersensitivity is lifelong).
2   Soothing soaks, such as diluted potassium permanganate (see Appendix II), are helpful.
3   Topical Grade I corticosteroids are prescribed and carefully monitored (see Appendix III).
4   Post-inflammatory hyperpigmentation is common, long-lasting and unaffected by treatment.

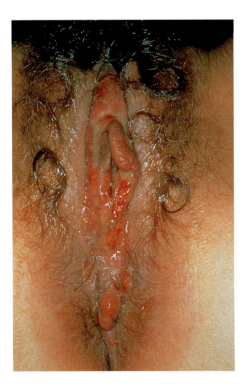

Figure 5.13
Fixed drug eruption. In this instance, the offending drug was co-trimoxazole.

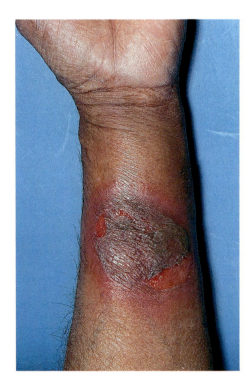

Figure 5.14
Fixed drug eruption. This case was also due to co-trimoxazole.

Bullous pemphigoid

Bullous pemphigoid is an uncommon auto-immune bullous disease which affects both skin and mucous membranes, usually in older women. Blisters form at the dermo-epidermal junction and thus are long-lasting and often haemorrhagic. A circulating autoreactive antibody can be found in the blood by an 'indirect' immunofluorescence technique using normal skin. The antibody can be demonstrated within lesions at the level of the dermo-epidermal site of blistering by 'direct' immunofluorescence techniques. Lichen sclerosus has been described in association with bullous pemphigoid as with other autoimmune diseases.

Management

1 The diagnosis is confirmed by biopsy and immunofluorescence (see Figures 2.9–2.11).
2 Local Grade I topical corticosteroids are prescribed and carefully monitored (see Appendix III).
3 In widespread cutaneous involvement, systemic treatment with oral cortico-steroids, often in combination with cytotoxics, is used. Specialist dermato-logical advice is required for the management of this condition.

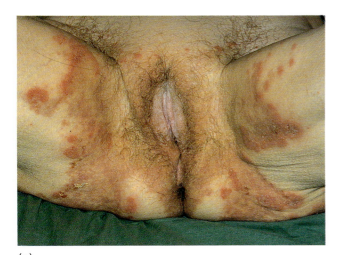

(a)

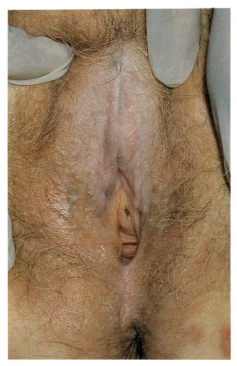

(b)

Figure 5.15
Bullous pemphigoid. (a) This 63-year-old lady with a 6-year history of lichen sclerosus, suddenly developed an intensely itchy and widespread bullous eruption on her body and perineum. Blistering is occurring on an intensely erythematous base, especially at the edge of the lesion. (b) Note the long-standing changes of lichen sclerosus which is seen better on this enlargement.

Pemphigus vulgaris

Pemphigus vulgaris is a rare severe immunologically mediated bullous eruption which affects mucous membranes and the skin. Blisters are fragile and seldom last long. A circulating autoreactive antibody can be found in the blood by an 'indirect' immunofluorescence technique on normal skin. The antibody can be demonstrated within lesions in the intercellular spaces (see Figure 5.19). Most patients are young adults.

Management

1   The diagnosis is confirmed by biopsy and immunofluorescence (see Figures 2.9–2.11).
2   Treatment of secondary infection can sometimes lead to remarkable improvement.
3   Local Grade I topical corticosteroids (see Appendix III) are sometimes better tolerated applied as a layer on alginate dressings when the lesions are eroded.
4   When large areas of skin are involved, systemic treatment with corticosteroids, often in combination with cytotoxics, is employed. Specialist dermatological advice is required for the management of this condition.

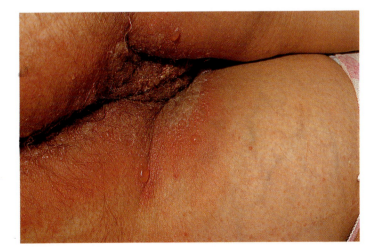

Figure 5.16
Blisters of pemphigus vulgaris.

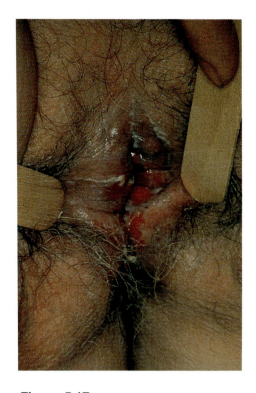

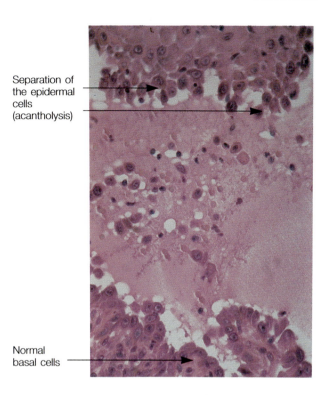

Separation of
the epidermal
cells
(acantholysis)

Normal
basal cells

Figure 5.17

A more typical presentation of pemphigus
vulgaris with erosions.

Figure 5.18

Histology of pemphigus vulgaris of the
vulva with acantholysis (arrow) (H & E,
×83).

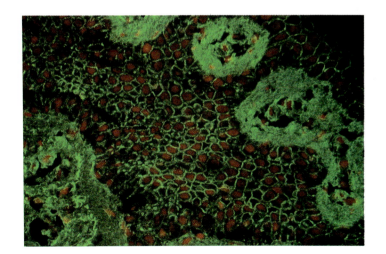

Figure 5.19

Pemphigus vulgaris. Direct
immunofluorescence showing
deposits of IgG and complement
in the intercellular spaces. The
titre of circulating pemphigus
autoantibodies can be measured
by an indirect immunofluorescence
test.

Pemphigus vegetans

Pemphigus vegetans is an extremely rare variant of pemphigus where hypertrophic verrucous lesions are formed during the healing phase, particularly in flexural areas.

Management

1 Careful search for secondary infection is important.

2 Wet compresses with diluted potassium permanganate can be very helpful (see Appendix II).

3 Grade I topical corticosteroids—sometimes better tolerated applied as a layer on alginate dressings—can be very helpful (see Appendix III).

4 Systemic steroids, with or without cytotoxic agents, may be required. Specialist dermatological advice is required for the management of this condition.

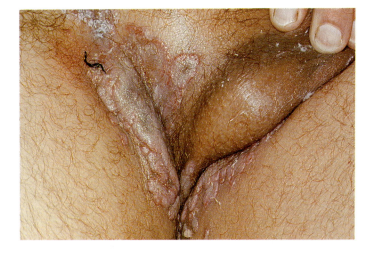

Figure 5.20
Pemphigus vegetans. The verrucous plaques are typical.

Cicatricial pemphigoid

Cicatricial pemphigoid is a very rare variant of pemphigoid in which mucous membrane involvement is the most prominent feature, and leads to scarring.

Management

1 A careful search should be made for secondary infection and appropriate treatment instituted.
2 Grade I topical corticosteroids are used spread thinly on alginate dressings (see Appendix III).
3 Sulpha drugs may be helpful, for example dapsone or sulphamethoxy-pyridazine (Lederkyn), which is only available on a named-patient basis for this indication. Care must be taken with these drugs because of their toxic side-effects.
4 Systemic steroids with or without cytotoxic drugs may be required. Specialist dermatological advice is required for the management of this condition.

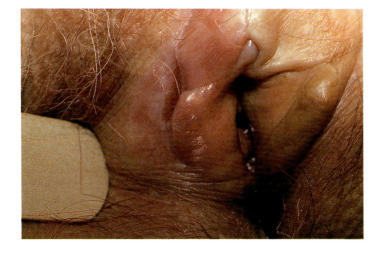

Figure 5.21
Cicatricial pemphigoid with vulval scarring.

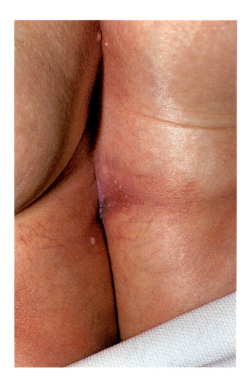

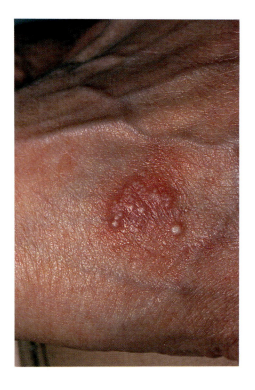

Figure 5.22
Cicatricial pemphigoid. Blisters on the posterior perineum have healed, leaving characteristic milia.

Figure 5.23
Cicatricial pemphigoid. The localized blister in the dorsum of the hand of the same patient as in Figure 5.22 has healed with milia formation.

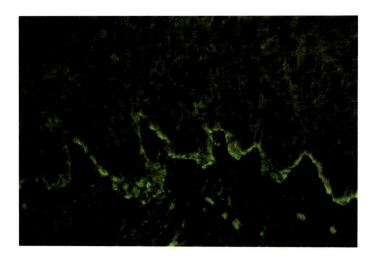

Figure 5.24
In cicatricial pemphigoid immunofluorescence may be positive, showing deposits of IgG at the dermo-epidermal junction.

Benign familial pemphigus (Hailey–Hailey disease)

Friction, occlusion and secondary infection are precipitating factors for blistering and erosions in this rare genetically determined disorder. Flexural areas are usually involved, including the vulva.

Management

1 The diagnosis is by punch biopsy (see Figures 2.9–2.11).
2 Bacterial secondary infection plays an important role in triggering exacerbations. Swabs should always be taken and repeated at regular intervals.
3 Reassurance of the benign localized nature of this condition is important.
4 Grade I topical corticosteroids with appropriate antibacterial treatment will often bring attacks under control; thereafter emollients alone, or Grade IV topical corticosteroids, may be enough to keep the condition under control (see Appendix III).

(a)

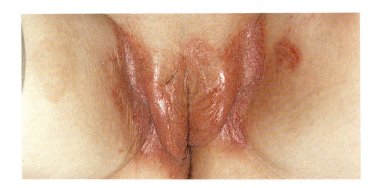

(b)

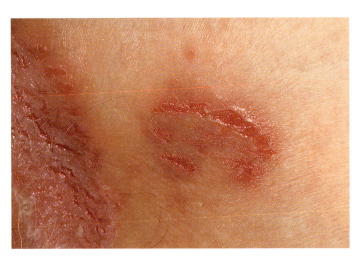

Figure 5.25
(a) Hailey–Hailey disease of the vulva and genitocrural folds.
(b) Enlargement shows the 'beefy-red' area on the vulva.

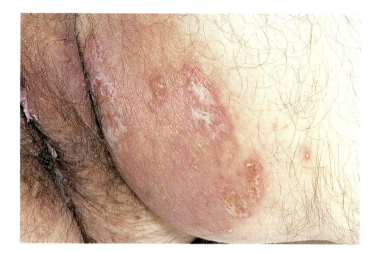

Figure 5.26
Hailey–Hailey disease. Close-up to show the transient blistering that may be seen in this disorder.

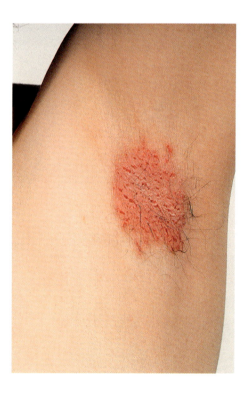

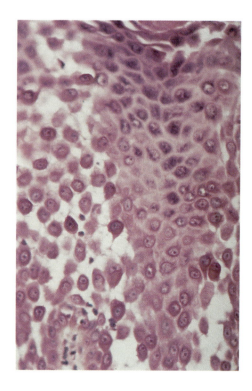

Figure 5.27
Hailey–Hailey particularly favours the great flexures, as seen here in the axillae.

Figure 5.28
Histology of vulval Hailey–Hailey disease. The epithelium has disintegrated, with acantholysis and clefting, giving a typical 'dilapidated brick wall appearance' (H & E, ×83). Immuno-fluorescence in these cases is always negative.

Darier's disease

Darier's disease is another genetically determined dermatitis characterized by waxy hyperkeratotic papules appearing in seborrhoeic areas. There may be involvement of the perineal skin.

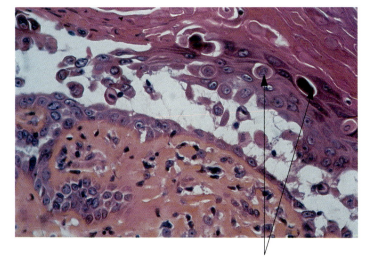

'Corps ronds'

Figure 5.29
Histology of Darier's disease. There is suprabasal clefting with acantholysis and 'corps ronds' (H & E, ×40). Immunofluorescence is always negative.

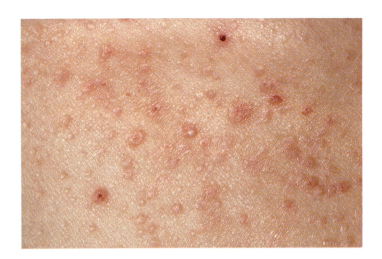

Figure 5.30
Darier's disease. Close-up view
showing follicular papules.

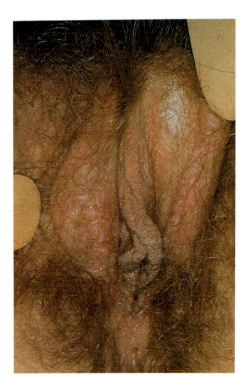

Figure 5.31
Darier's disease on the vulva. Here the horny
papules have coalesced to form moist plaques.

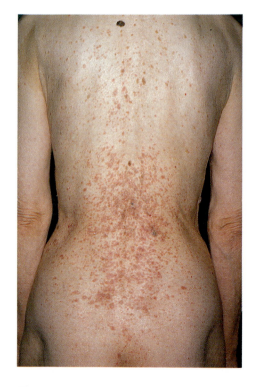

Figure 5.32
Typical Darier's disease on the back.

Necrolytic migratory erythema

A dramatic and recognizable pattern of spreading painful periorificial skin lesions can be due to an underlying glucagon-secreting pancreatic tumour. Necrolytic migratory erythema is extremely rare. Blood glucagon levels will be very high and there will be an accompanying anaemia, diabetes and a sore, 'beefy-red' tongue.

Management

1 Somatostatin subcutaneous injections are the mainstay of treatment. Advice from specialist centres should be sought.
2 Zinc and essential fatty acid infusions have helped some patients, but advice from specialist centres should be sought.

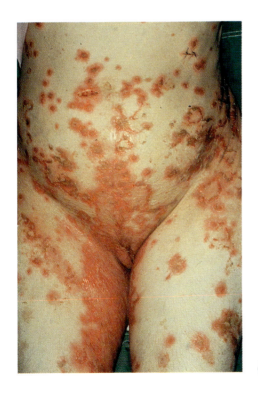

(a)

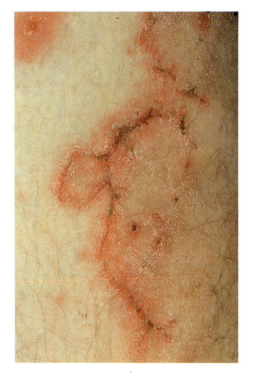

(b)

Figure 5.33

(a) Necrolytic migratory erythema. (b) A close-up view shows serpiginous eroded advancing edges.

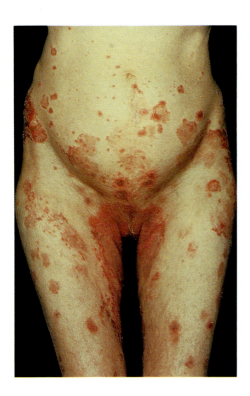

Figure 5.34
Necrolytic migratory erythema in a patient with pancreatic glucagonoma.

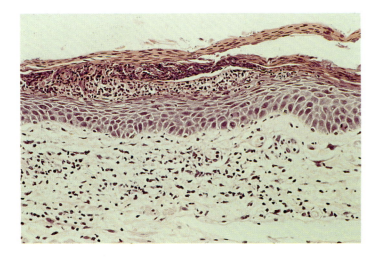

Figure 5.35
Histology of necrolytic migratory erythema. There is upper epidermal necrolysis with inflammatory cell infiltrate and overlapping parakeratosis.

Crohn's disease

Crohn's disease is not uncommonly accompanied by perineal ulceration and fistula formation. In rare instances, the only abnormality is chronic unexplained oedema of the vulva, as in the patient illustrated in Figure 5.36. This ectopic manifestation of Crohn's disease can be seen in all ages, even children.

Management

1 If the intestinal Crohn's disease is active, then therapy should be directed towards controlling this; often, the vulval ulceration will also improve.
2 If the Crohn's disease is not active elsewhere, local measures can be taken, such as potassium permanganate soaks (see Appendix II) and Grade I topical corticosteroids.
3 If involvement is severe and extensive, systemic steroids are necessary.

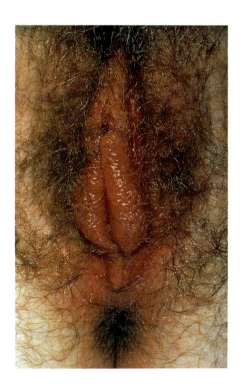

Figure 5.36
Crohn's disease. This patient presented with unexplained chronic vulval oedema.

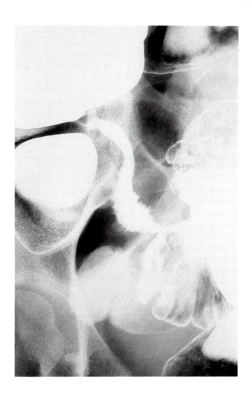

Figure 5.37
Crohn's disease (same patient as Figure 5.35). Barium enema shows narrowing of the terminal ileum, with 'thorn-like' crypts, which is typical of Crohn's disease. After abdominal surgery and oral steroids, her vulval oedema receded.

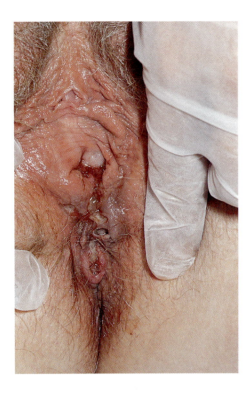

Figure 5.38

Crohn's disease. Extensive perineal ulceration with multiple fistulae. After failed medical treatment, total colectomy and ileostomy was curative.

6 Pilosebaceous inflammation

The adnexal structures of the labia majora include the pilosebaceous unit, but the labia minora have modified sebaceous glands where there is no associated hair follicle.

Epilation folliculitis (pili incarnati)

Shaving or plucking of the hairs in the 'bikini-line' may cause problems. Re-growing hair has a tendency to curl back on itself and may grow into normal skin, eliciting a marked foreign-body response with chronic purulent inflammation.

Management

1 Explanation of condition and reassurance are the basis of treatment.
2 Use of keratolytics after epilation may be helpful, e.g. 0.01% retinoic acid gel (beware local irritant effect).
3 Electrolysis is the only method that can permanently destroy the hair follicle and, though expensive, may be worth pursuing in some patients.

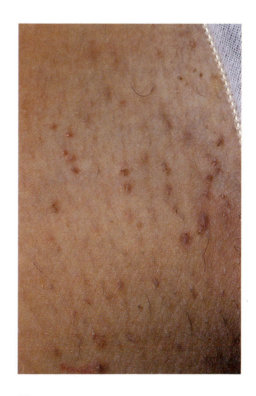

Figure 6.1
Epilation folliculitis.

Apocrine acne (hidradenitis suppurativa)

Acne of the apocrine gland-bearing areas causes deep perifollicular purulent inflammation sometimes forming interconnecting deep sinuses and abscesses. The characteristic early physical sign is the bridged comedone. Patients are usually in their twenties and often have a history of severe cystic acne.

Management

1 In the early stages, antiseptics and antibiotics may minimize purulent inflammation and scarring. Swabs should always be taken. Gram-negative and Gram-positive organisms may be found, often resistant to antibiotics recently used. Topical metronidazole can be helpful.

2 Hormonal treatment with anti-androgens, e.g. cyproterone acetate either in low dosage in a combined contraceptive pill (Dianette)—or with additional dosage (e.g. 25–50 mg daily) on days 5–15 of the cycle. Pregnancy must be avoided because of the feminizing influence on a developing male fetus.

3 Oral retinoids may be helpful, but teratogenicity limits their use in women of childbearing age.

4 Surgical excision of affected areas can be undertaken in those patients with very localized disease, or in cases with extensive disease recalcitrant to medical treatment.

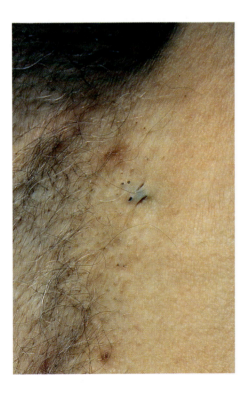

Figure 6.2
Apocrine acne with 'bridged' comedone.

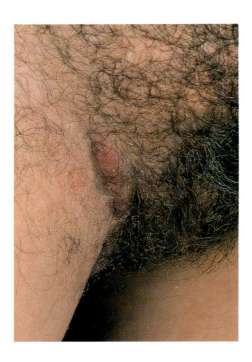

Figure 6.3
Line of typical apocrine acne nodules in the
inguinal crease.

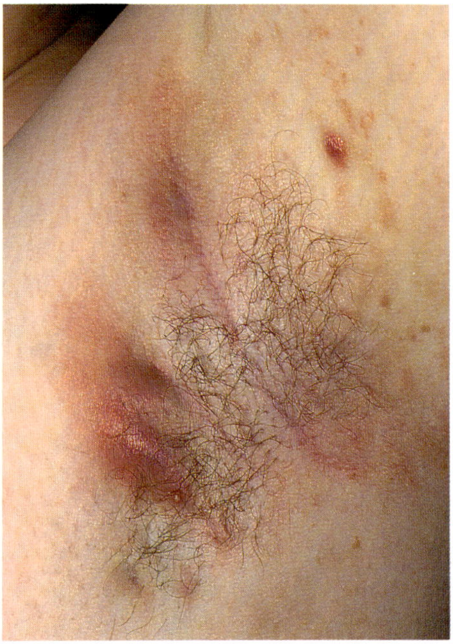

Figure 6.4
More extensive axillary involvement with
apocrine acne.

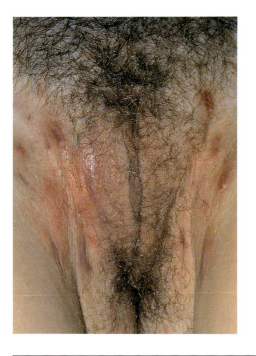

Figure 6.5
Hidradenitis suppurativa in a 25-year-old woman.

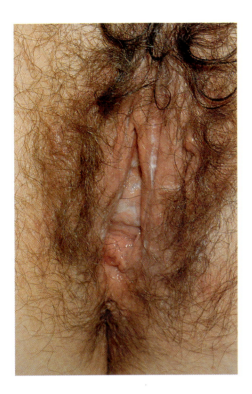

Figure 6.6
Apocrine acne.

7 Infections and infestations

The skin of the vulva harbours a wide population of microorganisms, particularly coagulase-negative staphylococci, lactobacilli and diphtheroids, with streptococci, coliforms and yeasts being noted in variable proportions in healthy women. Vaginal secretions contain epithelial cells, cervical glandular secretions and numerous streptococci and *Bacteroides* species are commonplace. *Ureaplasma urealyticum* and *Mycoplasma hominis* can both be found in healthy women, although debate continues about their association with particular conditions such as bacterial vaginosis or pelvic inflammatory disease. However, it is clear that neither viruses nor *Chlamydia trachomatis* are part of the normal vaginal or vulval flora.

Pathogenic infections of the vulva may reach this area via contamination from the patient's own skin, especially hands, via spread from the anus during defaecation or sexual contact. It is important to recognize that sexual contact may involve a variety of skin-to-skin or skin-to-mucous membrane contacts between the woman and her sexual partner. Sexually transmitted conditions, such as syphilis, chancroid, gonorrhoea and the chlamydial infections, and viral infections such as genital warts and herpes must be accurately diagnosed and differentiated from conditions such as candidiasis and bacterial vaginosis, which may be provoked or aggravated by sexual intercourse.

FUNGAL INFECTIONS

Candida albicans

Vaginal candidiasis is extremely common, presenting with a thick white discharge which causes maceration and irritation of the vulva. It often occurs following courses of antibiotics, during pregnancy, and in women taking the combined oral contraceptive pill. The cardinal symptoms are vaginal discharge with pruritus. Other commonly reported symptoms include dysuria and dyspareunia. Some 50% of women will attempt self medication prior to consulting a physician about such symptoms. The efficacy of the variety of home remedies used is unknown, but antiseptics, douches and assorted 'natural' remedies can significantly alter and/or exacerbate the clinical picture.

It is unusual for candida to infect the non-mucosal surfaces of the vulva, but if this does occur, diabetes should be excluded.

The diagnosis of vulvo-vaginal candidiasis is confirmed by microscopy and/or culture of vaginal secretions, but treatment should be initiated on the history.

Management

1   Treatment is usually local, by an imida-
    zole (e.g. clotrimazole pessaries or
    intravaginal cream).
2   More severe or recurrent infections
    require systemic therapy, with a 1-day
    course of a triazole such as itraconazole
    or fluconazole.
3   Although candidiasis is not a sexually
    transmitted condition, it can co-exist
    with other STDs.
4   Severe or recurrent vaginal candidiasis
    should prompt investigation to exclude
    diabetes mellitus or other causes of
    immunosuppression.
5   Information is most usefully given to the
    patient as a leaflet.

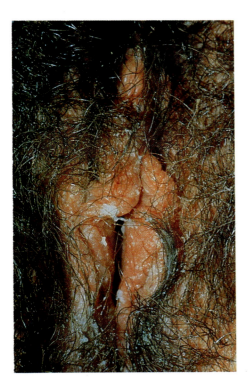

Figure 7.1
Vulvo-vaginal candidiasis. Note the red,
swollen labia and creamy discharge.

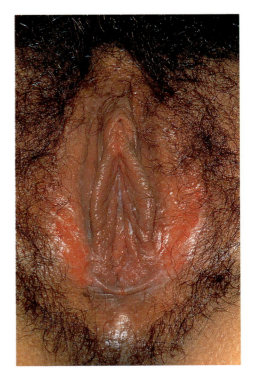

Figure 7.2
Erosive vulval candidiasis.

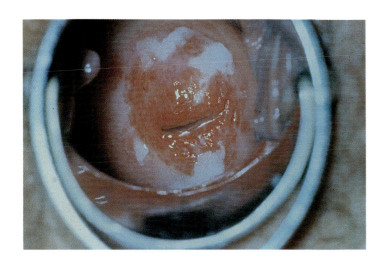

Figure 7.3
Cervical and vaginal candidiasis.

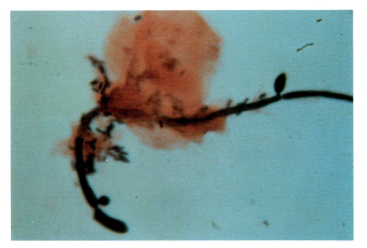

Figure 7.4
Gram-stained smear showing *Candida albicans*.

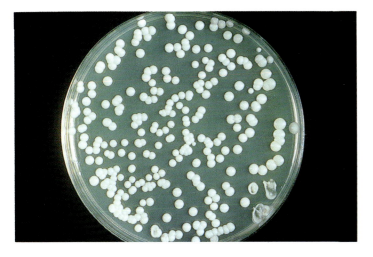

Figure 7.5
Culture of *Candida albicans* on Sabouraud's medium.

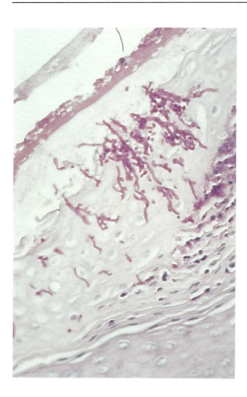

Figure 7.6
Histology of candidiasis. There are obvious pink-red hyphae in the stratum corneum (PAS, ×25).

Tinea infections

Dermatophyte infections of the crural area are mostly caused by *Trichophyton rubrum*. Vulval involvement in healthy adults is rare. Diagnosis is by skin scrapings which should reveal hyphae (see Figure 7.9), and culture yields the responsible dermatophyte fungus.

Management

1 If the vulva is acutely inflamed, potassium permanganate compresses are used (1 in 10 000) (see Appendix II).
2 A topical antifungal, e.g. clotrimazole or terbinafine cream, is prescribed.
3 If hair-bearing areas are involved, oral griseofulvin or terbinafine is the treatment of choice (e.g. griseofulvin 500 mg twice daily or terbinafine 250 mg daily, continued for one week after apparent cure).

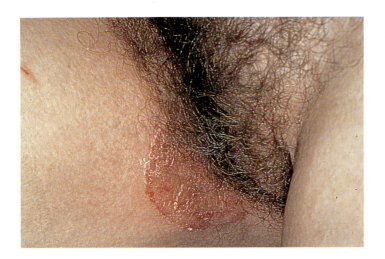

Figure 7.7
Tinea cruris. The fungus induces
inflammation at the advancing
edge of the lesion, so-called 'edge
activity'.

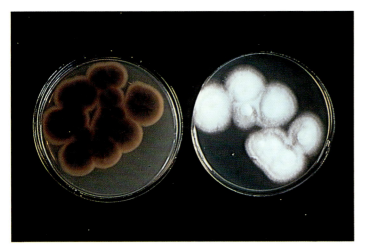

Figure 7.8
Trichophyton rubrum growing on
Sabouraud's medium.

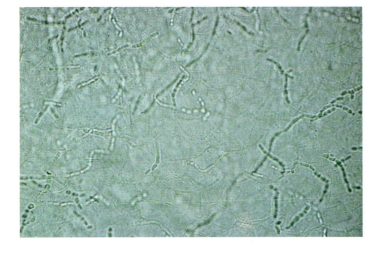

Figure 7.9
Hyphae of *Trichophyton rubrum* in
skin scrapings mounted in
potassium hydroxide
(H & E, ×40).

VIRAL INFECTIONS

Herpes simplex

Vulval herpes simplex is a common sexually transmitted genital infection. It may be acquired from either oral or genital lesions of a sexual partner but many cases have now been described in which the source partner is asymptomatically transmitting the virus. The reported incidence of genital herpes has increased over the past decade, but sero prevalence studies of those attending genitourinary medicine clinics have demonstrated that there is a considerable degree of underdiagnosis, with as many as 35% of attendees having evidence of previous HSV-2 infection which is undiagnosed. Herpes simplex virus (HSV) is a DNA virus with two subtypes, HSV-1 and HSV-2. Incubation period is usually between 3 and 10 days.

Previous exposure to either strain of herpes at another site gives some protection against severe primary genital infections. This is due to cross-reactivity between neutralizing antibodies present in the serum. The severity of symptoms and signs of primary genital herpes are greatest in those patients who have not previously been exposed to HSV (either 1 or 2) at any site. In such individuals, the local genital ulceration is painful and often extensive and is usually associated with both local and systemic complications. These can include fever, myalgia, meningism, draining lymphadenopathy and urinary retention (especially in women with extensive periurethral ulceration).

Patients with primary genital herpes require prompt systemic antiviral treatment as well as analgesia, bed rest and treatment of any secondary infection. Recurrent episodes are often managed by simple measures such as local hygiene and saline washing, but in patients with severe or frequent recurrences, investigation for underlying immunosuppressing conditions should be performed in conjunction with consideration of the options of episodic or continuous preventative systemic antiviral therapy.

Although the diagnosis of genital herpes is often made clinically, it is important to try to confirm this by culture or antigen testing. The patient's need for counselling and information about their diagnosis can often be best provided by specialists, for example in a genitourinary medicine clinic such as those in the UK. Although the majority of vulval herpes simplex infections recur 2–3 times per year or less, significant numbers of patients will be concerned about the risk of transmitting their infection to current or future sexual partners and will require specific supportive management to prevent their becoming demoralized or suffering psychosexual difficulties.

Management

1 Genital herpes simplex infection is usually sexually acquired, and it is vital to screen for other sexually transmitted infections (STIs).

2 There is an epidemiological but not causative link between genital herpes and the risk of cervical neoplasia. Women should be encouraged to participate in national cervical screening programmes.

3 Diagnosis is usually made by viral culture or an antigen test. The use of electron microscopy to examine vesicle fluid or a Tzanck smear stained with Giemsa to show typical multinucleate giant cells may be used in specialist centres. Furthermore, there is increasing availability in research centres of type-specific serological tests (such as Western Blot) to differentiate between Type-1 and Type-2 infections. These serological tests may be helpful in cases where diagnosis is difficult, or in counselling and advising sexual partners about the risk of infection.

4 Severe primary infection requires systemic antiviral treatment. The options for this are aciclovir 200 mg five times daily for 5 days, valaciclovir 500 mg b.d. for 5 days or famciclovir 250 mg b.d. for 5 days. Rarely, patients require admission to hospital for intravenous therapy. Patients will also require analgesia, bed rest and treatment of any secondary infection.

5 Patients with intermittently recurrent, mildly symptomatic genital herpes will require information about simple measures to dry lesions, such as saline washing or potassium permanganate soaks. Discussion with the patient about triggers which they have identified that prompt recurrences can be helpful.

6 In patients with severe or frequently recurring attacks of genital herpes, or those with severe psychosexual problems following their diagnosis, consideration should be given to either patient-initiated episodic therapy (e.g. famciclovir 125 mg b.d., valaciclovir 500 mg b.d. or aciclovir 200 mg 5 times daily for 5 days) or suppressive continuous preventative therapy with aciclovir.

7 Patients should be informed that asymptomatic shedding of the virus can occur from the genital tract and that this has been reported to result in transmission from asymptomatic patients to their sexual partners.

8 Patients with severe or very frequent lesions should be examined and investigated for evidence of other systemic disease and immunodeficiency.

9 Patients with genital herpes can become depressed and relationships may suffer following a diagnosis. The awareness of physicians about this and the provision of psychosexual support and counselling is an important part of management.

10 No formal contact tracing of patients presenting with genital herpes is required. However, in many cases the patient's partner wishes to be seen to discuss their partner's diagnosis and the issues of transmission to them.

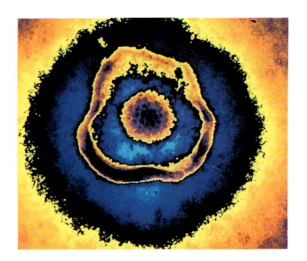

Figure 7.10

Herpes simplex virus. Colour-enhanced electron micrograph: the icosahedral protein capsid can be seen. This surrounds a core composed of double-stranded DNA.

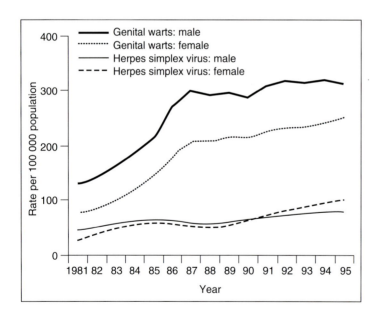

Figure 7.11

The incidence of genital herpes amongst GU clinic attenders has increased in recent years.

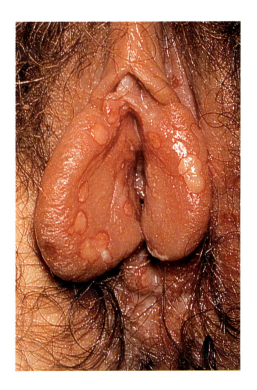

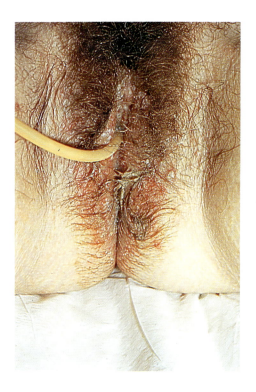

Figure 7.12

Primary genital herpes simplex virus infection of the vulva.

Figure 7.13

Severe primary vulvo-vaginal herpes infection, complicated by retention.

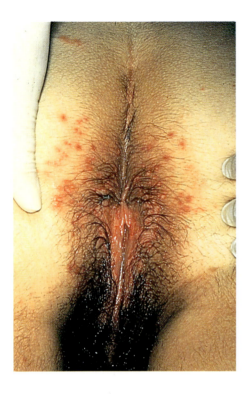

Figure 7.14
Perianal lesions of primary genital herpes.

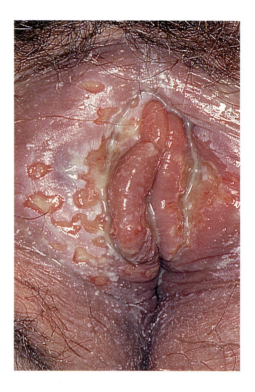

Figure 7.15
A severe primary herpes simplex infection with marked labial oedema.

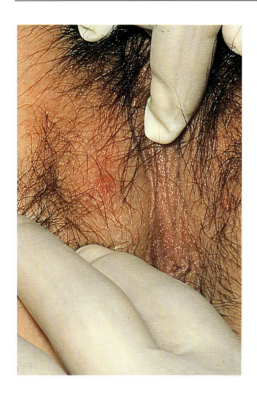

Figure 7.16
Recurrent genital herpes of the vulva.

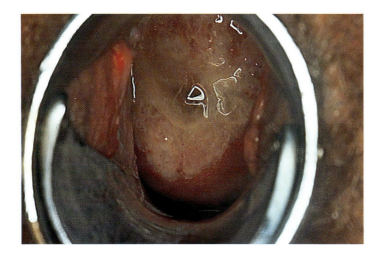

Figure 7.17
Acute erosive herpetic cervicitis.

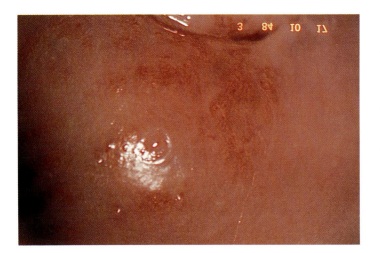

Figure 7.18
This colposcopic view of the cervix shows asymptomatic herpes shedding from the cervix. This patient had four lesions which were culture-positive for HSV. The majority of these episodes are accompanied by inguinal lymphadenopathy, dysuria or an increase in vaginal discharge.

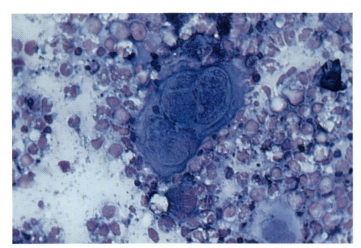

Figure 7.19
Tzanck smear of herpes showing multinucleated giant cells (Giemsa, ×50).

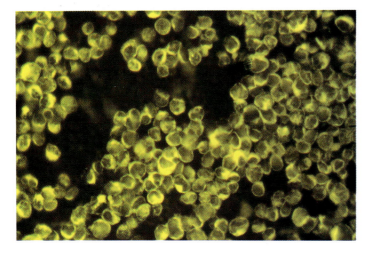

Figure 7.20
Smear stained by monoclonal immunofluorescent antibodies against HSV 2 (×40).

Recurrent varicella zoster virus (VZV) infection

Recurrent VZV infection, or shingles, is largely a disease of older patients. It represents the reactivation of the varicella zoster virus, which was acquired by the individual when they had chicken pox, often many years before. Rarely, when the S1, S2 and S3 dermatomes are affected, vulval skin will be involved, with the typical haemorrhagic vesicles. Frequent repeated episodes of shingles or multidermatomal disease should prompt investigation of the patient's underlying immunity.

Management

1 Potassium permanganate compresses are helpful (see Appendix II).
2 Topical silver sulphadiazine cream is prescribed.
3 Adequate analgesia is important.
4 It may be necessary to prescribe systemic antiviral therapy, such as aciclovir, famciclovir or valaciclovir, depending on the severity, the duration of lesions at presentation and whether there is risk of dissemination.
5 The patient should be followed up for possible post-herpetic neuralgia.

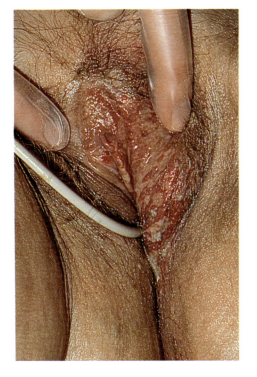

Figure 7.21
Severe vulval VZV infection.

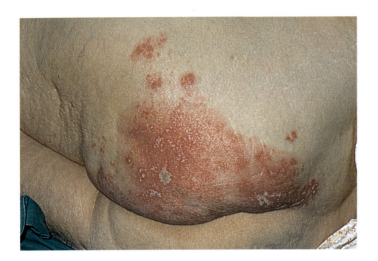

Figure 7.22
VZV infection affecting the buttock of the patient in Figure 7.21, showing unilateral distribution of the rash.

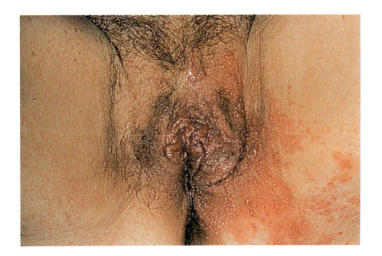

Figure 7.23
VZV infection of the vulva and buttock. Note the typical groups of vesicles. Prompt presentation and early antiviral treatment may reduce the subsequent risk of post-herpatic neuralgia.

Molluscum contagiosum

Molluscum contagiosum are small, hard infectious papules caused by a DNA pox virus. They thrive on atopic skin and may also be sexually transmitted. They grow rapidly and produce dome-shaped skin papules with central umbilication. Their natural history is usually spontaneous resolution within a 2-year period. However, in patients who are immunocompromised, spontaneous resolution does not always occur and the lesions may be very atypical in that they may be giant and atypically profuse.

Management

1 Any method of physical removal can be used (e.g. cryotherapy, curettage, extirpation or accurate phenolization). Pain can be minimized by applying a topical anaesthetic beforehand.
2 The patient should be reassured of eventual spontaneous resolution.

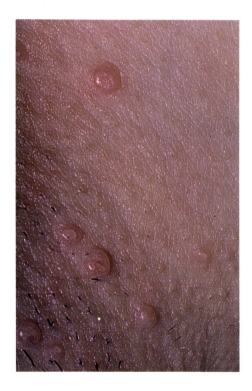

Figure 7.24
Molluscum contagiosum. Typical umbilicated papules of varying size.

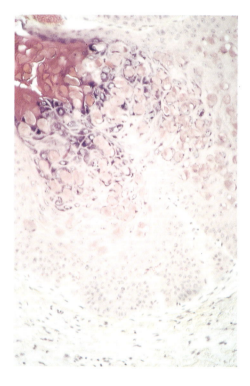

Figure 7.25
Histology of molluscum contagiosum. There is typical ballooning of keratinocytes and eosinophilic inclusion bodies (H & E, ×11).

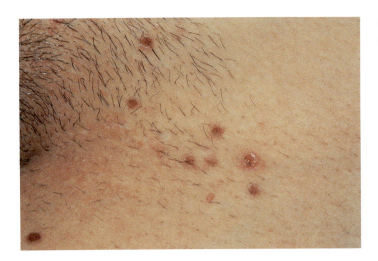

Figure 7.26
Peri-vulval molluscum contagiosum.

Warts—human papilloma virus infection

Genital warts are caused by infection with human papilloma virus (HPV). In all there are over 50 subtypes of virus. Genital warts are the most rapidly increasing STD. The presentation of this condition is most usually made by the patient themselves discovering they have lesions on their genitalia. However, in as many as 30% of cases, the diagnosis is made either because a partner develops lesions, or a physician examining the woman for another reason, notices lesions inside the lower genital tract. Although the diagnosis of HPV infection can usually be made clinically, it is important to recognize that there are differential diagnoses. These include condylomata lata of secondary syphilis, benign or malignant squamous tumours, as well as normal variants of vulvo-vaginal development. The oncogenic role of certain strains of these viruses is unclear in the aetiology of vulval carcinoma. In vulval carcinoma only some 30% of cases can be linked to virus, usually HPV 16 or 18.

Examination of the cervix visually (with the aid of the magnifying properties of a colposcope if available) and taking regular cervical cytology is indicated in cases of women presenting with intravaginal and cervical wart virus infection. The application of 5% acetic acid to the upper vagina and cervix can reveal areas of uncomplicated wart virus infection as well as the presence of dysplasia. All suspicious lesions should undergo biopsy to examine for the presence and degree of this cervical pre-neoplasia.

Patients with immunodeficiency may be very resistant to treatment and systemic treatments sometimes used include interferon. Treatment may be prolonged because of new lesion formation. Smoking seems to reduce the response to treatment.

Management

1 Although vulval warts are benign, they are sexually acquired and so it is important to screen for other sexually transmitted infections. This is probably best done in a GU clinic. Reassurance and conservative management should be an option made available to the patient. It must be made clear that sexual activity is likely to result in the transmission of HPV; therefore, in sexually active individuals, treatment and removal of lesions prior to resuming unprotected sexual intercourse should be advised.

2 If the patient has not had a cervical smear in the past 3 years, or is uncertain, a smear should be performed. If this is normal then she should be advised to ensure that she participates in a regular cervical screening programme. No extra cervical screening is required.

3 Warts can be removed by either physical or chemical methods:

A Physical methods include cryotherapy, which may need to be repeated on 2 or 3 occasions before lesions resolve. Diathermy or hyfrecation often require local anaesthetic, as does curettage. In some centres laser ablation is available; this also requires local anaesthesia.

B Physical methods are preferred for internal lesions and for all lesions in women who are, or may be, pregnant. Chemical methods include Podophyllotoxin, applied twice daily by the patient herself for three days each week until lesions resolve. This may be in the form of a solution or, in new preparations, a cream, which spreads less and carries less inflammation to surrounding skin.

C Podophyllin or trichloroacetic acid needs to be accurately painted on by a doctor or nurse and must be washed off 2–3 hours later. This treatment is usually repeated once- or twice-weekly.

D Interferon has been used as an adjunct to physical treatment or by itself. Intralesional injections appear to be efficacious but the expense and side effects mean that this should be reserved for treatment-resistant cases.

E Inosine pranobex (Imunovir) is a biurnal adjunctive therapy for genital warts at a dose of 1 g tds for 14–28 days. There is no data that adjunctive immunotherapy has any effect on reducing the likelihood of recurrent lesions.

F Intralesional injection of 5-fluorouracil is now licensed in several countries and, despite its cost, may be of value in the treatment of cases resistant to topical physical or chemical methods.

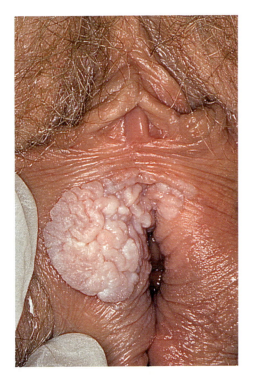

Figure 7.27
Vulval human papilloma virus infection.

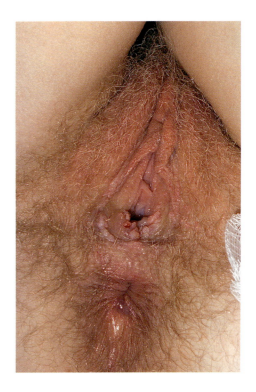

Figure 7.28
Vulval and perianal viral warts. Note the
uniform pink colouring.

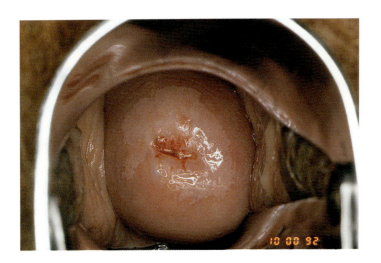

Figure 7.29
Flat subclinical wart virus infection
of the cervix.

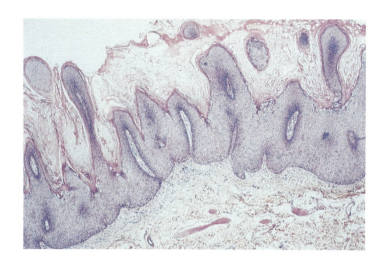

(a)

Figure 7.30

Histology of vulval warts. (a) There is hypertrophy of the epithelium, with acanthosis and papillomatosis showing confluent rounded rete pegs (H & E, ×11). (b) Enlargement shows maturation of epithelium without nuclear atypia. Koilocytic cells are seen in the upper layers (H & E, ×40).

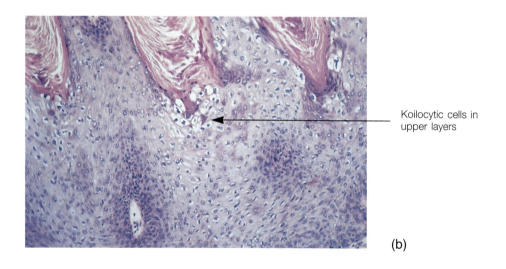

Koilocytic cells in upper layers

(b)

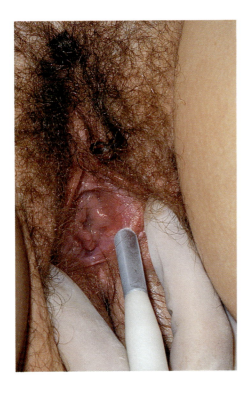

Figure 7.31
Vulval human papilloma virus infection
undergoing cryotherapy.

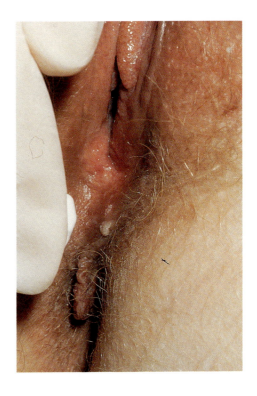

Figure 7.32
Application of podophyllotoxin cream to a
vulval wart. For prolonged use, the patient can
be given a latex glove to protect her finger
from inflammation.

Figure 7.33
Diathermy of vulval warts.

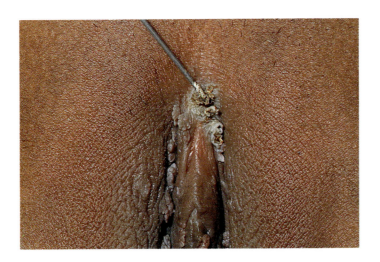

INFESTATIONS

Lice

The body and head louse (*Pediculus humanus*) does not affect the vulval area; the louse responsible for affecting this area is the crab louse (*Phthirus pubis*). The incubation period of *P. pubis* is 30 days. Crab lice need frequent blood feeds and are unable to survive for more than 24 hours away from their hosts.

Patients usually present with intense pruritus or may observe movement in their pubic hair. This is nearly always a sexually transmitted problem. Pubic lice may also be found on axillary, or more rarely, eyelash hair. The scalp is hardly ever affected.

Management

1 Aqueous malathion lotion (0.5%) is applied to all hairy areas except the scalp for 24 hours.
2 The patient is instructed to wash bed linen and clothes at a temperature above 50°C.
3 A second application of aqueous malathion is only necessary for heavy infestation. Shaving hair off is unnecessary.
4 Screening for other STDs and of contacts is carried out.

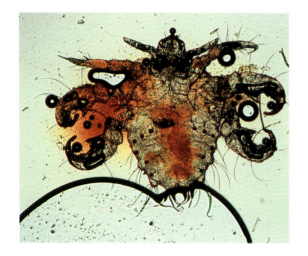

Figure 7.34

Phthirus pubis, the crab louse, is 1–2 mm long with three pairs of legs. The back legs are especially developed for grasping hairs.

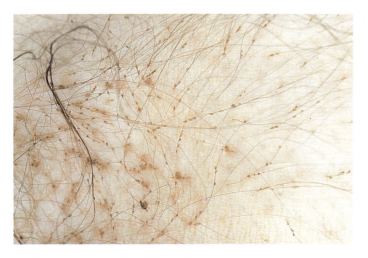

Figure 7.35
(a and b) Pubic hair showing infestation with crab lice.

(a)

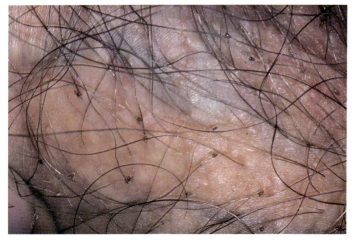

(b)

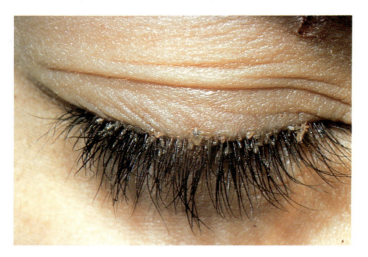

Figure 7.36
Crab lice on eyelashes.

Scabies—*Sarcoptes scabiei*

Scabetic infestation of the vulva is extremely rare. It causes a widespread and intensely pruritic skin eruption. Transmission of scabies requires prolonged intimate contact between individuals.

Management

1 It is essential that all close contacts of the patient are treated simultaneously.
2 Treatments include aqueous lindane (1%), aqueous malathion (0.5%) and 5% permethrin cream. Usually one treatment is sufficient, but if necessary it can be repeated.

BACTERIAL INFECTIONS

Staphylococci

These ubiquitous organisms occasionally cause infections of the vulva which may be misdiagnosed as STDs such as herpes. The areas of inflammation are often centred on the hair follicle and may follow cosmetic depilation or other causes of trauma.

In bartholinitis, patients present with painful unilateral vulval swellings. The cause is an obstruction of the long duct to Bartholin's glands which are sited deeply.

Management

1 The organisms should be cultured and their sensitivity determined.
2 Diabetes or other general medical conditions must be excluded.
3 Pili incarnati should be excluded (see Figure 6.1).
4 Topical antiseptics and antibiotics are applied.
5 Systemic antibiotics such as flucloxacillin (e.g. 250–500 mg four times a day for 5 days) may be required.

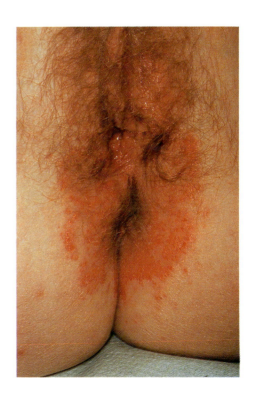

Figure 7.37
Bacterial impetigo of the perineum.

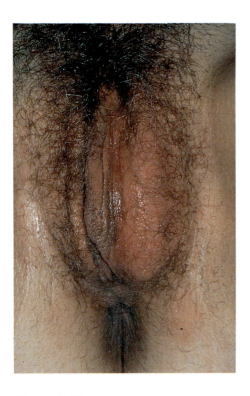

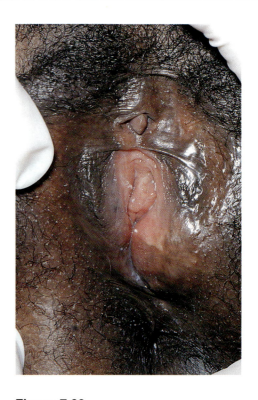

Figure 7.38

Acute staphylococcal bartholinitis. In this case,
surgical marsupialization was necessary.

Figure 7.39

Acute bartholinitis. Again, surgical
marsupialization was performed.

Gonorrhoea

Gonorrhoea is caused by *Neisseria gonorrhoeae*. Although the incidence of gonorrhoea in men declined significantly in the mid 1980s, the rates of infection in women declined less dramatically. These reductions were believed to be due to the more widespread use of condoms and the practice of less penetrative sexual intercourse following publicity about AIDS. As 70% of women with anogenital gonococcal infection are asymptomatic at the time of diagnosis, it is important to contact trace the partners of index patients who are diagnosed as having this infection. In women, the infection primarily involves columnar epithelium in the endocervix and the urethra. It must be remembered that oropharyngeal and anal infections can occur in people who have used these sites sexually. Ascending infection can result in endometritis, salpingitis with the sequelae of infertility, ectopic pregnancy and pelvic pain. Rarely, gonococcal septicaemia can result in arthritis and discrete purulent skin lesions. Involvement of the vulva is rare, but the gonococcus can infect the Bartholin's gland, resulting in abscess formation.

Management

1 This is a sexually acquired disease and patients should be screened for other STDs. This is probably best done in a GUM clinic.
2 Ampicillin is the drug of choice, given with probenecid (e.g. ampicillin 3 g as a single oral dose and probenecid 1 g as a single oral dose).
3 Penicillin-hypersensitive individuals can be treated with ciprofloxacin (500 mg orally immediately).
4 Treatment failures may be due to re-infection or resistant organisms. Ciprofloxacin or spectinomycin can be used (e.g. spectinomycin 2 g injected intramuscularly). Contact tracing and screening for other STDs must be carried out.

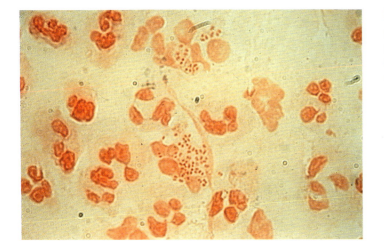

Figure 7.40

Neisseria gonorrhoeae appearing as intracellular Gram-negative diplococci on this Gram stain of endo-cervical smear.

Syphilis

The causative agent in syphilis is *Treponema pallidum*. Its incidence has been decreasing over the past decade in developed countries. However, over the past 3 years, urban centres in America have reported a dramatic increase in the cases of both primary and secondary syphilis in heterosexual men and women, as well as a dramatic increase in the incidence of congenital syphilis. Syphilis is a venereal disease and remains the great mimicker of other conditions. Although it produces florid signs of a primary chancre and, later, the classic lesions of secondary, tertiary and quaternary syphilis, syphilis can only be diagnosed during its latent phase by serological tests. In view of the recent increase in cases in the USA, as well as the important interaction of syphilis in increasing the risk of acquisition and transmission of HIV, it is vital that serological surveillance is maintained of sexually active people at risk of acquiring syphilis.

Management

1   This is a sexually acquired disease and patients should be screened for other STDs. This is probably best done in a GUM clinic.
2   Treatment is penicillin, given intramuscularly for 10 days (e.g. 1.2 mega-units injected intramuscularly daily for 10 days).
3   Individuals who are hypersensitive to penicillin should be treated with doxycycline (e.g. doxycycline 100 mg twice daily orally for 21 days).
4   Serological follow up after treatment is mandatory to ensure evidence of effective therapy.
5   Contact tracing of sexual partners is essential.

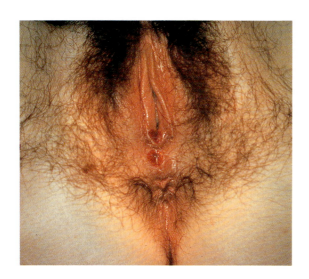

Figure 7.41

Syphilis – primary chancre. This begins as a small papule which rapidly ulcerates. The incubation period is 9–90 days. There is always draining non-tender lymphadenopathy.

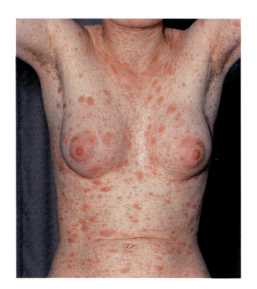

Figure 7.42

Secondary syphilis. Typical 'messy' papolosquamous eruption. The patient was unwell with sore throat, headaches and lymphadenopathy.

Erythrasma

A common bacterial infection of warm, moist folds, erythrasma is more common in the tropics, in obese patients and in diabetics. The organism, Corynebacterium minutissimum is a short, gram-positive rod which requires special media for culture.

Infection may be asymptomatic or may cause considerable itch, with reddish-brown macular patches spreading out from the flexures. The central clearing and edge activity of fungal infections is not seen. Examination of the patient in a dark room with an ultraviolet (Wood's) lamp reveals characteristic coral-pink fluorescence.

Management

1   Diagnosis confirmed by Wood's light examination.
2   Scrapings for bacteriological culture on special medium.
3   A topical antibiotic, e.g. 2% clindamycin solution or 2% miconazole cream, should be applied.
4   A systemic antibiotic may be required, e.g. erythromycin 250 mg q.i.d. for 6 days.
5   Relapse is common, especially in diabetics. Glycosuria should be ruled out.

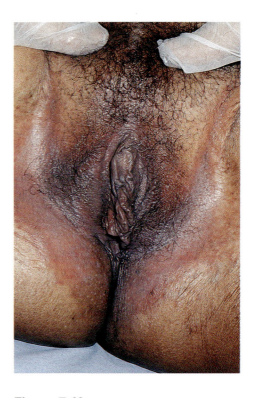

Figure 7.43

Erythrasma affecting the labia majora and crural folds of this 40-year-old black woman. This would show up as a fluorescent, coral pink under Wood's light.

Chancroid

Chancroid is caused by *Haemophilus ducreyi*. It is a rare STD in Europe and even rarer in women. It occurs mostly in Africa, Asia and South America.

Three to ten days after exposure small papules appear and break down to form tender non-indurated ulcers. Unilateral lymphadeno-pathy occurs in a half of patients and such glands may eventually rupture.

Management

1 This is a sexually acquired disease and patients should be screened for other STDs. This is probably best done in a GUM clinic.
2 Treatment is co-trimoxazole or erythromycin for 7–10 days (e.g. co-trimoxazole 960 mg twice daily or erythromycin 500 mg four times a day).

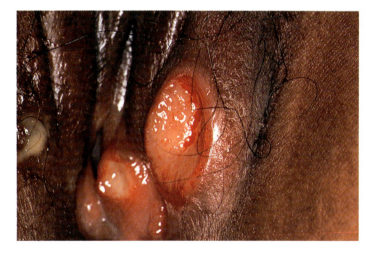

Figure 7.44
Vulval chancroid.

Reiter's syndrome and sexually acquired reactive arthritis (SARA)

The classic triad of arthritis, urethritis and conjunctivitis constitute Reiter's syndrome. SARA is a term used to relate to the arthritis following a suspected genitourinary infection, though it does accommodate extra-genital and extra-articular manifestations. The characteristic cutaneous features seen with Reiter's syndrome are keratoderma blenorrhagica and, in men, circinate balanitis. Keratoderma blenorrhagica most commonly affects the soles of the feet and may spread to the dorsum, genitalia, palms, trunk and scalp. It initially appears as brown macules and then progresses to heaped-up lesions with scaling, resulting in an appearance histologically identical to that seen in psoriasis. Ungual involvement may result in nail plate dystrophy and in a fifth of cases ulceration has been reported in the oral cavity.

Although the male/female ratio of incidence is approximately 20:1, this probably reflects the higher likelihood of asymptomatic genitourinary infection occurring in women and thus a relative under-diagnosing of this association. Caucasians are at greater risk than blacks, this relationship being independent of the rate of HLAB27 positivity.

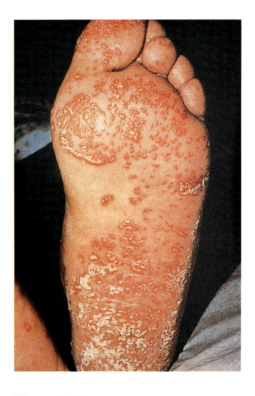

Figure 7.45
Keratoderma blenorrhagia. Typical 'barnacle-like' eruption on soles of feet.

Management

1   Management is aimed at eradicating the infectious aetiology with standard treatment for chlamydial infection where indicated.
2   Local cutaneous manifestations can be managed as for psoriasis (see page 45).
3   In cases of severe joint involvement, systemic steroids or agents such as azathioprine may be indicated.

Lymphogranuloma venereum

Lymphogranuloma venereum is a largely tropical STD caused by *Chlamydia trachomatis*. After an incubation period of 10 days, a painless lesion may develop in the vagina, which heals rapidly and is usually unnoticed. Three to four weeks later, lymphadenopathy develops. Chronic anogenital infection may lead to fistulae, which may later be complicated by carcinomatous change.

Management

1 This is a sexually acquired disease and patients should be screened for other STDs. This probably best done in a GU clinic.
2 Treatment is oxytetracycline or erythromycin for 2–3 weeks (e.g. oxytetracycline 250 mg four times a day or erythromycin 500 mg four times a day).
3 Surgical treatment of complications of untreated disease.

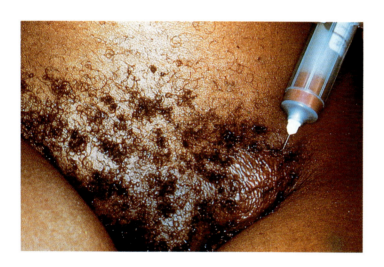

Figure 7.46
Lymphogranuloma venereum. Syringe aspiration of swelling in the left groin showing purulent, blood-stained contents.

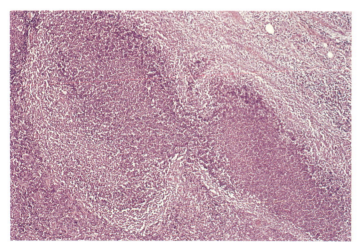

Figure 7.47
Histology of lymphogranuloma venereum.

Bacterial vaginosis

The diagnosis of bacterial vaginosis is made by the presence of a malodorous greyish discharge of pH ⩾ 5, which shows a positive amine test and the presence of clue cells on microscopy of a Gram stain smear. The cause of this discharge is a mixed vaginal infection, by *Gardnerella vaginalis* and an aerobic organism (especially *Bacteroides* species and *Mobiluncus* species). There is no evidence that this infection is sexually transmitted although it is more common in sexually active women. It should be suspected in women with malodorous vaginal discharge which is exacerbated by sexual activity and causes marked vulvo-vaginal pruritus.

Management

1 No treatment is required in women who are asymptomatic.
2 In those with symptoms, treatment is either oral metronidazole 400 mg twice daily for 5 days, or vaginal application of clindamycin 2% cream daily for 7 days.
3 The avoidance of local irritants to the vagina and vulval areas is recommended.
4 Unfortunately, up to 40% of women will develop recurrent episodes; more efficacious long-term therapies are currently being evaluated, including the use of vaginal acidifying agents such as Aci-jel (Cilag).
5 In pregnant women, bacterial vaginosis has been linked to an increased risk of preterm delivery. Treatment of asymptomatic women may be beneficial in this situation.

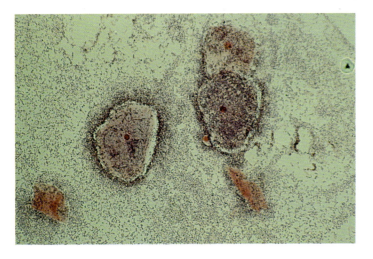

Figure 7.48
Bacterial vaginosis. Microscopic appearance of Gram-stained slide from vaginal discharge, demonstrating a clue cell. This is an epithelial cell covered by diverse types of micro-organism to produce a classic 'salt and pepper' appearance (×150).

PROTOZOAL INFECTIONS

Vaginal trichomoniasis

Trichomonas vaginalis is a motile flagellate protozoan which causes a malodorous profuse greyish-green frothy vaginal discharge. This causes vulval irritation and erythema. It is usually sexually transmitted, although waterborne infection can occur.

Diagnosis is by microscopic examination of a wet smear. Culture on Whittington–Feinberg medium is useful in difficult cases.

Management

1 Vaginal trichomoniasis is usually a sexually acquired disease and patients should be screened for other STDs, particularly gonorrhoea. This should be done in a GUM clinic.
2 Treatment is metronidazole or nimorazole (e.g. metronidazole 400 mg twice daily for 5 days, or nimorazole 2 gm at once orally) or topical therapy with clindamycin, 2% gel.
3 It is usual to treat the male partner.
4 Increasing numbers of cases of metronidazole-resistant trichomoniasis have been reported. Laboratory confirmation and exclusion of sexually acquired reinfection are important. New therapies urgently need to be evaluated.

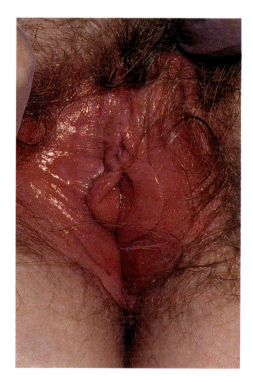

Figure 7.49
Trichomoniasis of the vagina. Gross primary irritation and oedema of the vulva, caused by severe vaginal trichomoniasis.

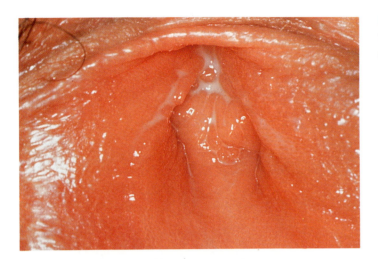

Figure 7.50
Trichomoniasis of the vulva
showing periurethral involvement.

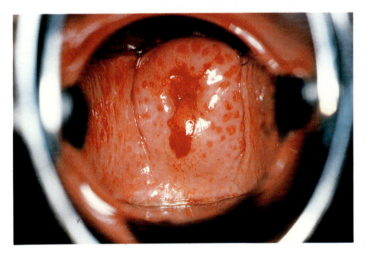

Figure 7.51
'Strawberry' cervix of severe
trichomoniasis.

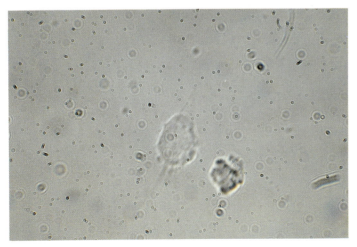

Figure 7.52
Trichomoniasis of the vagina,
diagnosed by microscopic
examination of a wet smear
(×100).

Helminth infestations

Vulval schistosomiasis

Schistosomiasis is caused by the human blood flukes *Schistosoma mansoni, S. japonicum* and *S. haematobium*. Vulval infection can result from swimming in lakes in endemic areas containing cercariae released from aquatic snails. These free-swimming cercariae rapidly penetrate human skin. After maturation in the liver, flukes pass into the pelvic veins and lay eggs which penetrate the rectum and bladder and hence may be voided. Some worms or ova may migrate through adjacent vasculature and cause subcutaneous granulomata especially in the peroneum, groin and external genitalia.

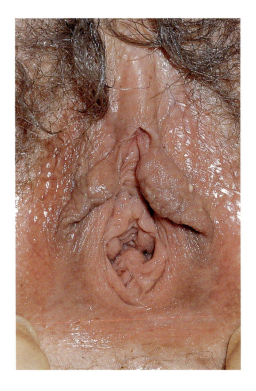

Figure 7.53
Vulval schistosomiasis. This 25-year-old caucasian woman presented with an uncomfortable enlargement of the left labia of 6-month duration, asking for surgical correction.

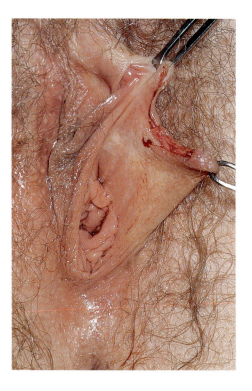

Figure 7.54
Operative view showing wedge of labia minora excised in 'V'.

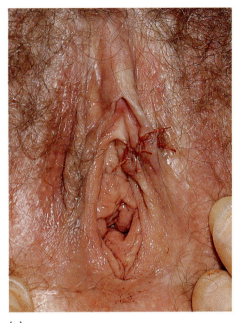

(a)

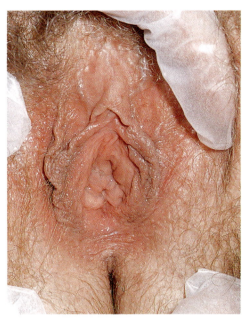

(b)

Figure 7.55

(a) Closure of wound with interrupted vicryl in two layers. The histological specimen showed vulval schistosomiasis! This is a rare condition confined to women who have swum in water contaminated by *schistosomiasis mansoni*, *japonicum* or

haematobium. The patient had swum in Lake Malawi eighteen months previously. (b) The same patient six weeks later, with good cosmetic and functional results.

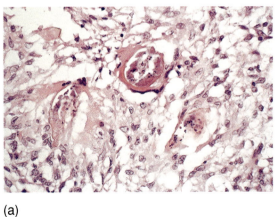

(a)   (b)

Figure 7.56

Schistosomiasis with calcified ova and giant cell reaction; (a) H&E, ×11, (b) H&E, ×40.

8 Tumours

Congenital tumours

The following examples of tumours are the ones most commonly seen in an out-patient clinic.

Capillary naevi present at birth and are permanent. There will be no functional sequelae and laser treatment depends on cosmetic considerations.

A strawberry naevus (cavernous haemangioma) is usually not present at birth but appears within the first 6 weeks of life, and sometimes grows rapidly. Lesions may cause problems early on because of this, with risk of secondary infection and, rarely, septicaemia. Lesions gradually resolve spontaneously over a 10-year period. Treatment should, therefore, be reassurance that the lesion will resolve.

Congenital phimosis of the clitoris is a rare developmental abnormality of the labia minora. Careful surgical dissection restores function and prevents the abscess formation that will otherwise occur.

Benign tumours

Any tumour can occur on the vulva. Those derived from adnexae will be largely confined to the labia majora, but histopathological analysis is essential for definitive diagnosis. The following are the most common lesions.

1 *Acrochordia (skin tags)*—these are common in all frictional or flexural sites such as axillae, eyelids and groins. They can achieve large size and torsion can lead to painful thrombotic infarction. Treatment is by scissor amputation.
2 *Venous varicosities*—these may become exaggerated during pregnancy and resolve after delivery. They rarely cause obstetric problems.
3 *Keratinous cysts*—multiple closed and open comedones. Similar lesions are often seen on the scrotum. Secondary infection or calcification can occur.
4 *Vestibular mucous cysts*—these arise anywhere within the vestibule and are harmless.
5 *Papillary hidradenomata*—these are the most frequent cutaneous adnexal tumours at this site. They present as small nodules and frequently ulcerate. They resemble pyogenic granulomata.
6 *Syringomata*—these very uncommon eccrine duct tumours present as asymptomatic papules of the labia majora and are usually multiple.

7 *Giant venous ectasia*—this is a dramatic and florid form of venous varicosity of the labia. Such lesions dilate further during pregnancy, and sometimes may be troublesome during delivery. Rarely, there can be underlying arterio-venous malformation.

8 *Haematocolpos*—this is an extremely rare tumour which presents at the introitus with a history of cyclical pain and primary amenorrhoea at the time of puberty. Treatment is by surgical incision, releasing typical dark, altered blood.

9 *Endometrioma*—this discrete papule presents as pain and swelling premenstrually.

10 *Prolapse of urethral mucosa*—this presents with an asymptomatic tumour.

Management

1 Keratinous cysts—these are best excised under local anaesthetic.

2 Papillary hidrandenomata—these require excision for histological examination.

3 Syringomata—biopsy may be required to make the diagnosis; extensive lesions can be treated by hyfrecation or electro-dessication.

4 Giant venous ectasia—surgical intervention can lead to alarming haemorrhage and many surgeons choose to leave such lesions (providing they are asymptomatic) untreated.

5 Haematocolpos—surgical incision to release typical dark, altered blood, and drainage with tampon insertions until the next period. Other developmental abnormalities of the genito-urinary tract should be excluded.

6 Endometrioma—biopsy may be required to establish the diagnosis. The lesions can be destroyed by excision laser therapy, but extensive or recurrent disease may require hormonal treatment to suppress ovulation (e.g. danazol 200–800 mg daily for three to six months or goserelin 3.6 mg subcutaneously over 28 days).

7 Prolapsed urethral mucosa—conservative treatment is preferable.

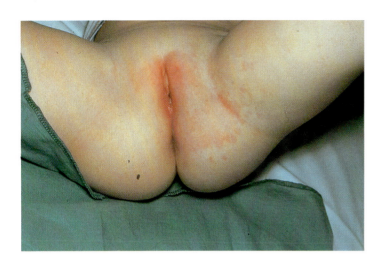

Figure 8.1
Capillary naevus.

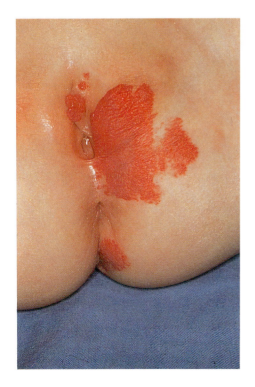

Figure 8.2
Strawberry naevus.

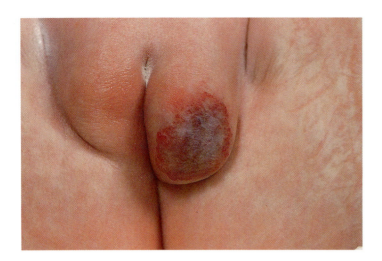

Figure 8.3
Strawberry naevus. This lesion was not present at birth, appeared at 6 weeks and grew quickly. In this photograph, at age 2½, the lesion is shrinking. Note the characteristic grey surface marking the involution phase. Conservative management is usually favoured unless urinary outflow is compromised.

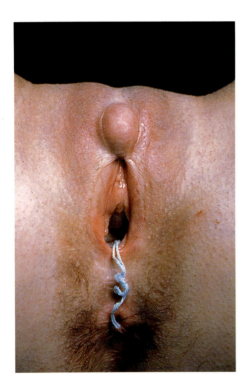

Figure 8.4
Congenital phimosis of the clitoris.

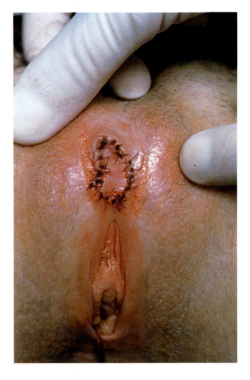

Figure 8.5
Surgical dissection of congenital phimosis.

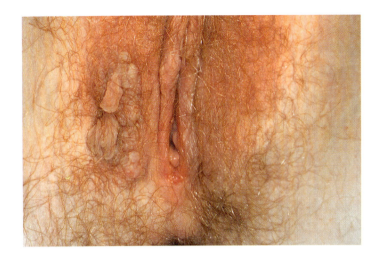

Figure 8.6
Acrochordia (skin tags).

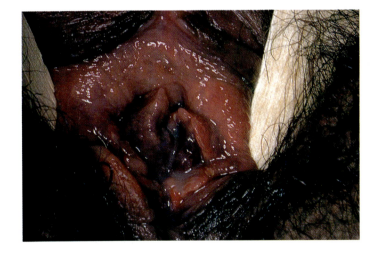

Figure 8.7
Vulvo-vaginal varicosities.

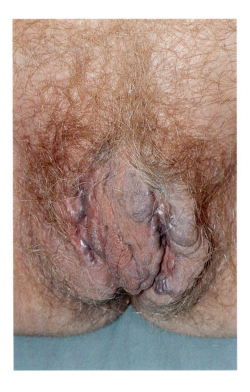

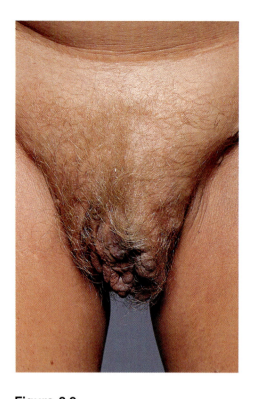

Figure 8.8

Extensive vulval varices in a 38-year-old primagravida at term.

Figure 8.9

The same patient as in Figure 8.8 standing, showing venous engorgement in inguinal area. Elective caesarian section was uncomplicated and was followed by shrinkage of varicosities.

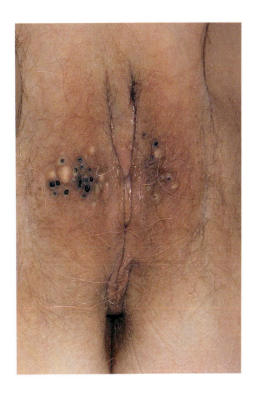

Figure 8.10
Keratinous cysts.

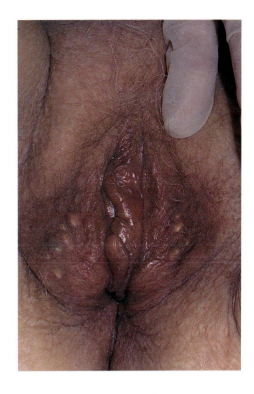

Figure 8.11
Multiple epidermoid cysts of labia majora.

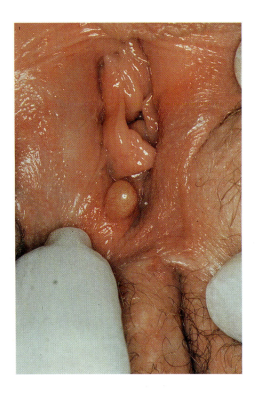

Figure 8.12
Vestibular mucous cysts.

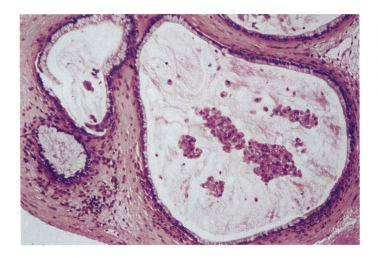

Figure 8.13
Vestibular mucous cyst—here, several cysts are seen lined by a single layer of columnar epithelium (H & E, ×40).

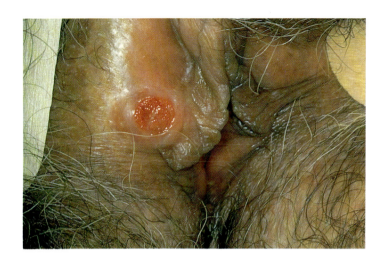

Figure 8.14
Papillary hidradenoma.

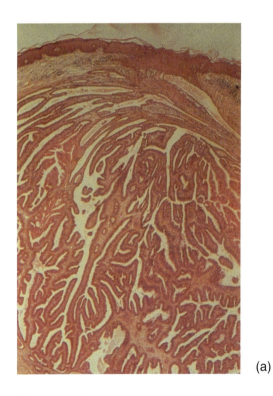

(a)

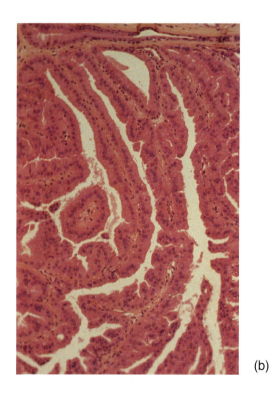

(b)

Figure 8.15

(a) Histology of papillary hidradenoma. There is a well-defined dermal tumour with proliferating tubular fronds (H & E, ×11).

(b) Enlargement shows two cell types reminiscent of apocrine tissue (H & E, ×40).

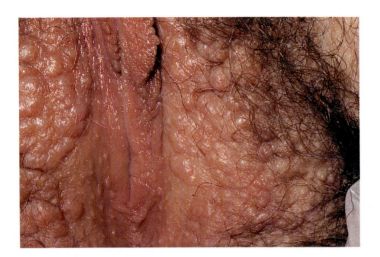

Figure 8.16
Syringomata.

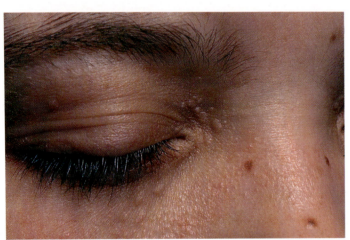

Figure 8.17
Syringomata at the more usual periocular site.

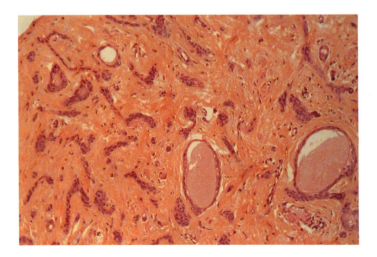

Figure 8.18
Histology of syringomata. There is proliferation of eccrine ductules in 'tadpole' shapes; some of the ducts have become blocked and show dilated cysts (H & E, ×40).

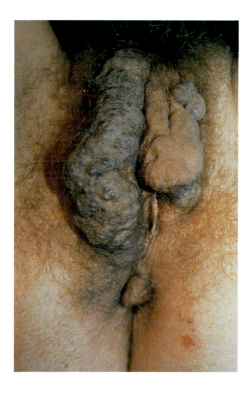

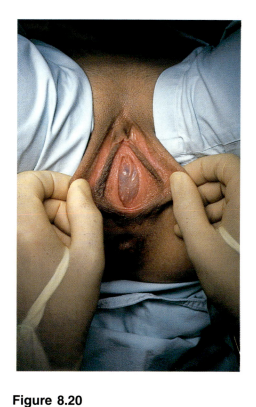

Figure 8.19

Giant venous ectasia of the labia. This patient did not turn out to have an underlying arterio-venous malformation, and spontaneous vaginal delivery following normal pregnancy occurred in her case.

Figure 8.20

Haematocolpos in a 13-year-old girl with a non-perforated hymen. The bluish swelling of the hymen is characteristic of an haematocolpos. After releasing the blood through an incision, the hymen has to be reconstructed.

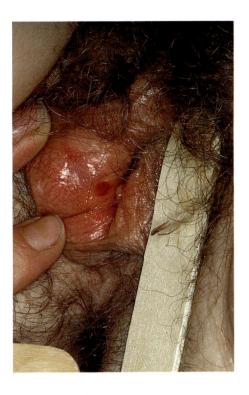

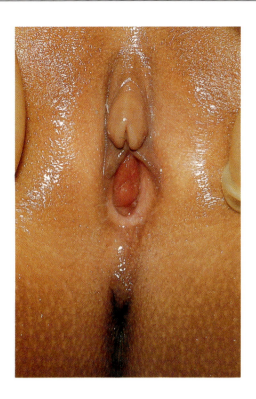

Figure 8.21
Endometrioma. Note the small discrete papule on the right labia minora.

Figure 8.22
Prolapsed urethral mucosa in a 9-year-old black girl. Conservative treatment is preferable.

9 Intra-epithelial neoplasia

There is understandable confusion about intra-epithelial neoplasia. Clinicians have perhaps tended to rely on the pathology report for a diagnosis. This is dangerous and can lead to mutilating overtreatment. As in most areas of dermatology, clinicopathological correlation is mandatory for a diagnosis. Clinically, the two most important points are:

- The age of the patient.
- Whether the lesions are single or multiple.

It is most important to realize that lesions with a benign evolution and those with malignant potential can be indistinguishable histopathologically. Only when squamous cell carcinoma occurs can a firm histological diagnosis be made. The term 'vulval intra-epithelial neoplasia, grade III' (VIN III; see classification on page 6) has been introduced to replace the older terms of bowenoid papulosis and Bowen's disease, both of which are described in more detail below.

Bowenoid papulosis

First described in the late 1960s, Bowenoid papulosis is predominantly a problem of young, sexually active women. It usually runs a benign course and spontaneous remission occurs in over 60% of cases. Clinically, there is a scattering of variously coloured 'stuck on' lesions at any site in the perineum. Most have a warty surface, but some can be smooth and shiny. Perianal involvement is very common. A large proportion of these patients have evidence of human papilloma virus infection of the cervix and need cervical smears. Anecdotal cases of micro-invasive disease have occurred in immunocompromised patients or those with very extensive lesions.

Management

1 Management is difficult, but is usually conservative, as the disease is multifocal and affects young women. Biopsy of any suspicious lesions is advisable, particularly of areas that show erosion or reddening.
2 Treatment by laser ablation is often disappointing, with high recurrence rates; local surgical excision, if practicable, is to be preferred.
3 Radical surgery, such as vulvectomy, is usually not indicated.
4 Long-term follow-up is essential as invasive disease can and does occur, although the incidence is low.

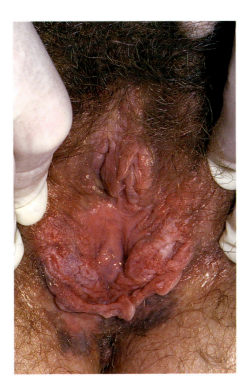

Figure 9.1
Bowenoid papulosis. There is diffuse involvement of the labia minora, posterior commissure and perianal area with extensive verrucous plaques. Note that some are white and some hyperpigmented. These lesions have a benign prognosis, but cervical smears should be taken.

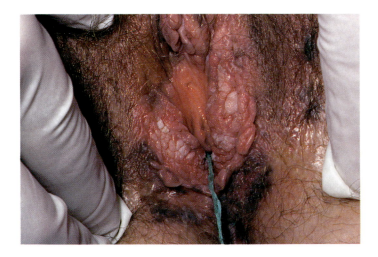

Figure 9.2

Bowenoid papulosis. Another patient showing a similar picture of extensive warty lesions of variable colour on the vulva and perineum.

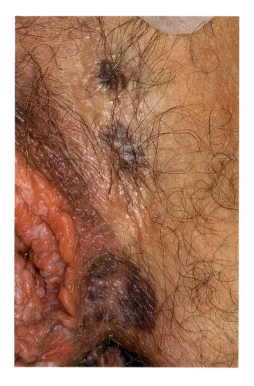

Figure 9.3

Bowenoid papulosis. Close-up view of the genito-crural fold showing pigmented seborrhoeic wart-like lesions.

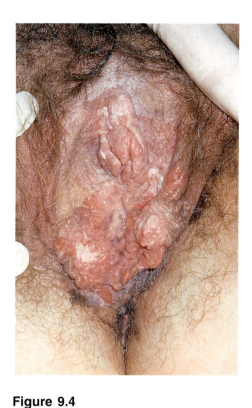

Figure 9.4

Florid Bowenoid papulosis. The whole of the vulva is covered in warty hyperkeratotic lesions, varying in colour, some areas being white, some red and some dark brown. The histology of such lesions is as in Figure 9.13. A case of extensive lesions like these should be followed up.

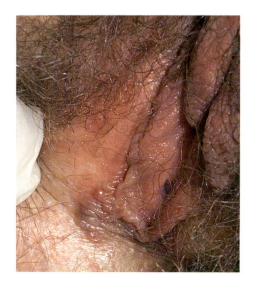

Figure 9.5

Bowenoid papulosis showing almost translucent pearly lesions in this patient.

Bowen's disease

Bowen's disease usually presents as a *solitary* plaque, and occurs in older women. Lesions may be white, red or pigmented and spontaneous remission does not occur. This type of solitary lesion should be removed by total excision. A proportion will progress to invasive squamous cell carcinoma.

Management

Possible methods of destroying an area of full thickness dysplasia include cryotherapy, diathermy, topical cytotoxics e.g. 5-fluorouracil, CO_2 laser (with or without interferon) and surgical excision. The precise plan for the management of any individual patient must depend on a variety of factors:

- *Age*—the older woman is more at risk of progressing to invasive disease.
- *Immune status*—those with immunodeficiency require more aggressive treatment.
- *Solitary lesion*—usually solitary lesions are more amenable to surgery.
- *Eroded and ulcerative lesions*—these must be biopsied adequately to exclude micro-invasive disease.

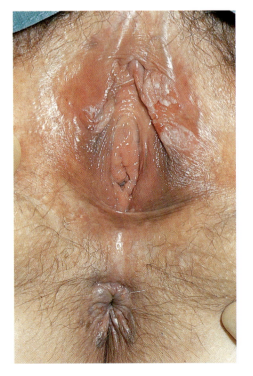

Figure 9.6

Multifocal Bowen's disease (VIN III) in a 35-year-old, which was highly symptomatic.

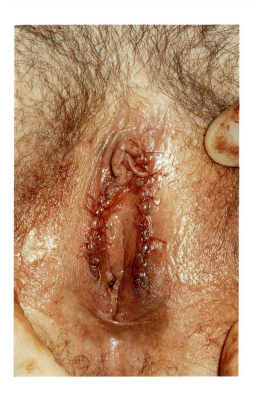

Figure 9.7
Wide local excision produced symptomatic relief and
no loss of vaginal function.

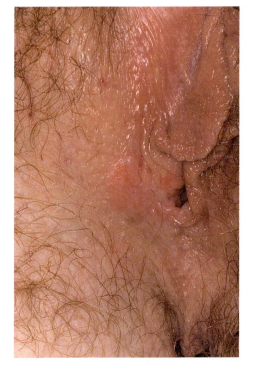

Figure 9.8
Bowen's disease. Note the contrast of this unifocal
reddened warty plaque at 7 o'clock.

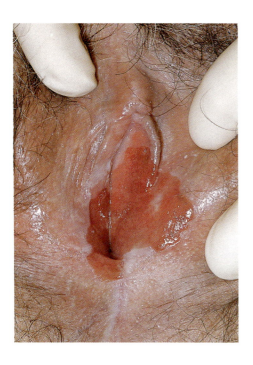

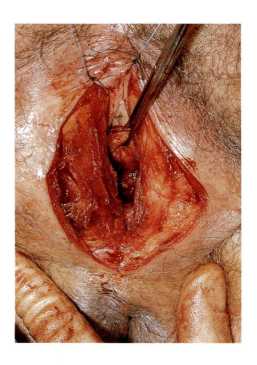

Figure 9.9
62-year-old woman with Bowen's disease (VIN
III). Note the characteristic well-demarcated
glassy red appearance.

Figure 9.10
Operative view showing simple vulvectomy.

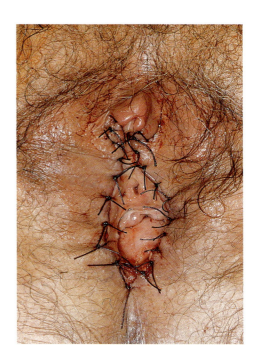

Figure 9.11
Operative view after closure. The eventual
cosmetic and functional result was satisfactory.

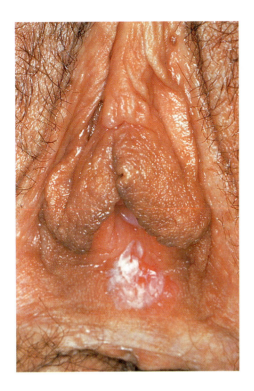

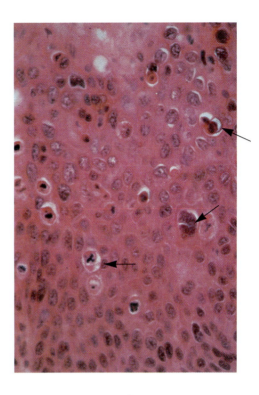

Figure 9.12

Bowen's disease. A solitary red plaque with a white warty surface, which in the past might have been referred to as 'leukoplakia'.

Figure 9.13

Full thickness atypia (VIN III). This type of full thickness atypia characterizes both Bowenoid papulosis and Bowen's disease; contrary to earlier teaching, the two conditions cannot be differentiated histologically (H & E, ×83). Arrows (→) show abnormal mitoses.

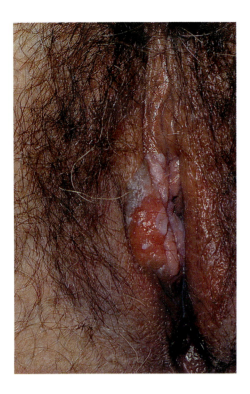

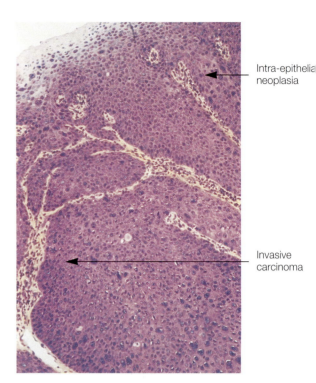

Figure 9.14

Bowen's disease progressing to invasive squamous cell carcinoma. This 60-year-old woman had a long-standing plaque of Bowen's disease which eventually progressed to this ulcerative eroded invasive tumour.

Figure 9.15

Histology of squamous cell carcinoma arising in Bowen's disease (same patient as in Figure 9.14). In the upper right hand corner, full thickness dysplasia can be seen. In the lower part of the photomicrograph, frank invasive squamous cell carcinoma can be seen protruding into the dermis (H & E, ×40).

10   Malignant disease

Malignant disease of the vulva is fortunately rare, representing only 3–5% of genital cancers. The average gynaecologist will only see one case a year. The majority of cases occur in women over the age of 60 who present with a long history of vulval irritation, pruritus, bleeding, pain, discharge or a lump. The mean delay in presentation is more than 10 months.

Aetiology

The aetiology is unclear. The majority arise on a background of lichen sclerosus. The remainder may be associated with full-thickness atypia (VIN 3) or arise de novo. Approximately 90% of tumours are squamous cell carcinomas (see Table 10.1).

The disease is more common in women with pre-existing genital tract neoplasia, e.g. cervical intra-epithelial neoplasia.

Staging of vulval carcinoma

The staging of vulval carcinoma is given in Table 10.2.

The staging of the disease before surgery continues to be unsatisfactory, with errors in at least 25% of cases. Palpation of groin nodes is notoriously difficult and in 20% of cases positive

Table 10.1 Histology of vulval tumours in 100 patients

Tumour	No.
Squamous carcinoma	90
(i) well-differentiated	52
(ii) moderately differentiated	23
(iii) poorly differentiated	15
Melanoma	6
Adenocarcinoma	2
Others, e.g. Bartholin's gland	2

Reprinted with permission from Grimshaw RM, Murdoch JB & Monaghen JM, Radical vulvectomy and bilateral inguinal-femoral lymphadenectomy through separate incisions – experience with 100 cases, *Int J Gynaecol Cancer* 1993; 3:18–23.

nodes may be impalpable. Lymphography is disappointing but fine needle aspiration and monoclonal labelling have yet to be properly assessed.

Intraoperative sampling and frozen section provide a better way of planning treatment, particularly in relation to the role of deep inguinal or pelvic node dissection.

Recent reports suggest that almost 50% of tumours are Stage I at presentation with similar proportions less than 2 cm in size. The majority of tumours are lateral, with approximately 25% affecting the clitoris.

Table 10.2 Staging of vulval carcinoma

Stage I	Lesions 2 cm or less confined to the vulva or perineum. No lymph node metastases.
Stage Ia	Lesions 2 cm or less in size confined to the vulva or perineum with stromal invasion no greater than 1.0 mm.* No nodal metastases.
Stage Ib	Lesions 2 cm or less in size confined to the vulva or perineum and with stromal invasion greater than 1.0 mm*. No nodal metastases. The more advanced stages are as previously defined.
Stage II	Tumour confined to the vulva and/or perineum or more than 2cm in the greatest dimension with no nodal metastases.
Stage III	Tumour of any size arising on the vulva and/or perineum with 1. adjacent spread to the lower urethra and/or the vagina or anus and/or 2. unilateral regional lymph node metastases.
Stage IVa	Tumour invading any of the following: upper urethra, bladder mucosa, rectal mucosa, pelvic bone and/or bilateral regional nodal metastases.
Stage IVb	Any distant metastasis including pelvic lymph nodes.

*The depth of invasion is defined as measurement of the tumour from the epithelial stromal junction of the adjacent most superficial dermal papilla to the deepest point of invasion.
Reprinted with permission from Shepherd JS, on behalf of Gynaecological Cancer Committee, International Federation of Gynaecology and Obstetrics. Cervical and vulval cancer; changes in FIGO definitions of staging. *B J Obstet. Gynaecol* (1996) **103**: 405–6.

Most authorities now accept the concept of microinvasive disease Stage Ia, otherwise known as 'superficially invasive vulvar cancer'. Pathologists differ in how they measure the depth of invasion, but most accept that it should be measured from the epithelial-stromal junction of the most superficial dermal papilla to the deepest point of the invasion.

Nodal involvement

Nodal involvement is common, even in early stages of the disease. A full understanding of this fact is essential for the optimum management of vulval cancer.

The relationship between nodal involvement, tumour size and depth of invasion is shown in Tables 10.3 and 10.4.

Table 10.3 Relationship between size of vulval carcinoma and groin node metastasis

Lesion size (cm)	Positive nodes (%)
<1	4.3
1–2	18.2
2–4	33.3
>4	53.3 (including pelvic nodes)

Reprinted with permission from Hacker NF et al, Management of regional lymph nodes and their prognostic influence in vulvar carcinoma. *Obstet Gynaecol* 1983; 61:408–12.

Table 10.4 Relationship between depth of invasion of vulval carcinoma and groin node metastasis

Depth of invasion (mm)	Positive nodes (%)
<1	0
1–5	11.6
5–7	42.9

Reprinted with permission from Hacker NF et al, Individualisation of treatment for Stage 1 squamous cell vulvar carcinoma. *Obstet Gynaecol* 1984; 63:155–62.

Table 10.5 Treatment of vulval carcinoma according to stage

Stage		Treatment	Approx. 5 year survival
1a	less than 1 mm invasion >8 mm margin	Wide local excision	>95%
1b	>1 mm laterally placed unifocal	Wide local excision + ipsilateral lymphadenectomy ± contralateral lymphadenectomy (if nodes positive)	95% (62%)
Ib	Central lesion	Radical vulvectomy + bilateral lymphadenectomy	90%
II		Radical vulvectomy + bilateral lymphadenectomy	85%
III & IV		Radical vulvectomy + bilateral lymphadenectomy ± chemotherapy and/or radiotherapy	50%
If tumour > 4 cm		Consider pelvic node dissection	

Treatment

Traditionally, invasive vulval cancer has been treated aggressively with the modified 'butterfly incision' combining radical vulvectomy and bilateral groin node dissection.

Although good results are obtained by this procedure, unacceptably high mortality and morbidity may follow. Prolonged immobilization, wound breakdown, thromboembolism, lymphoedema, bladder and sexual dysfunction are not uncommon.

Treatment should be planned and managed by an integrated team headed by a gynaecological oncologist. Surgery is tailored according to the individual woman and will depend on her age, fitness, tumour size, invasion, staging, sexual function and other factors. The trend is towards less aggressive surgery in women with early stage lateral disease, with a consequent reduction in morbidity and no reduction in cure rates (see Table 10.5).

Good results may be obtained by a three-incision technique, avoiding the traditional 'butterfly incision'.

Overall 5-year survival is 60% (corrected for intercurrent disease it is 75%); 92% survive if the nodes are negative and 31% if positive.

Management

1 Best managed by an experienced gynaecological oncology team including surgeons, pathologists, counsellors, nurses etc.
2 Care can be individualized according to tumour staging, size, position and nodal involvement.
3 Clinical staging can be misleading—nodal metastases may not be palpable.
4 Nodal involvement is very rare if invasion is less than 1 mm.
5 Early lateral tumours can be managed by wide local excision with ipsilateral node dissection in certain cases.
6 Early central lesions and all stage II, III and IV lesions should be managed by radical vulvectomy and bilateral lymphadenectomy.

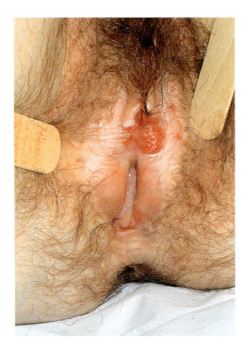

(a)

Figure 10.1

(a) Squamous cell carcinoma arising in lichen sclerosus.

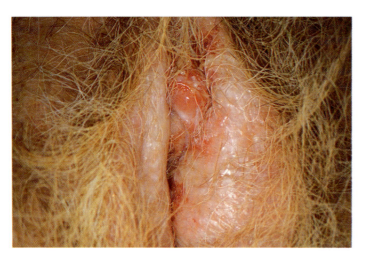

(b) Note the periclitoral site of the tumour. The lichen sclerosus shows extensive white spot disease and purpura.

(b)

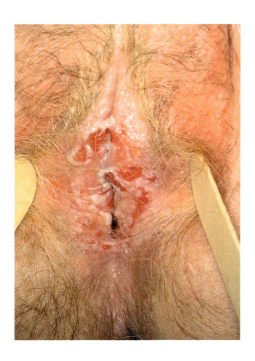

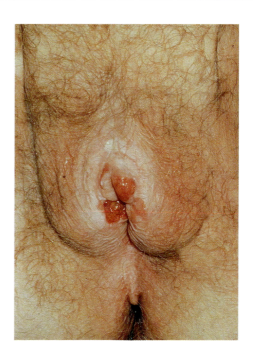

Figure 10.2

Multicentric squamous cell carcinomas arising in lichen sclerosus.

Figure 10.3

Squamous cell carcinoma — note background lichen sclerosus.

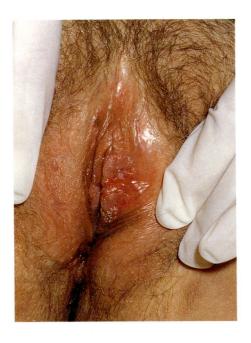

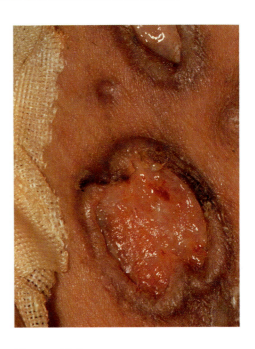

Figure 10.4
Squamous cell carcinoma arising in a younger woman without clinical or histological lichen sclerosus.

Figure 10.5
Squamous cell carcinoma showing multiple metastases in perineal skin.

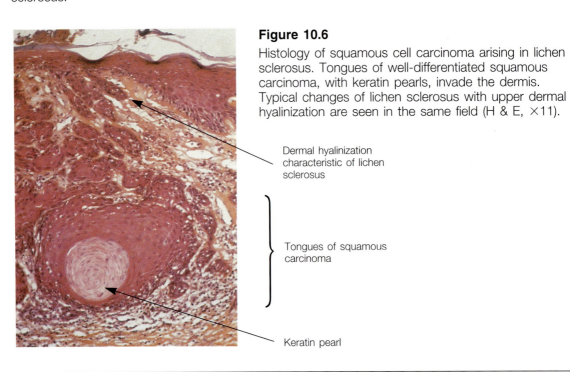

Figure 10.6
Histology of squamous cell carcinoma arising in lichen sclerosus. Tongues of well-differentiated squamous carcinoma, with keratin pearls, invade the dermis. Typical changes of lichen sclerosus with upper dermal hyalinization are seen in the same field (H & E, ×11).

Dermal hyalinization characteristic of lichen sclerosus

Tongues of squamous carcinoma

Keratin pearl

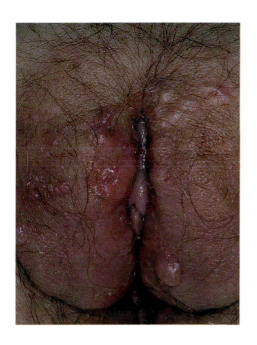

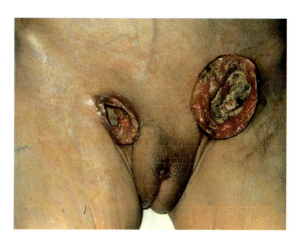

Figure 10.8
Ulcerative metastatic inguinal disease.

Figure 10.7
Vulval lymphangiectasia. This case was secondary to carcinomatous lymph node· obstruction.

Verrucous carcinoma of Buschke–Löwenstein

These rare tumours occur on vulval skin and produce alarming cauliflower-like lesions. They have been reported in association with papilloma virus infection and in some cases have arisen on a background of lichen sclerosus. They have well demarcated edges and extend deeply into the vulva. There is a remarkable separation between the tumour and surrounding normal tissue.

The histology is often very banal and the diagnosis can be missed if it has not been suggested clinically. This tumour should not be confused with a well-differentiated squamous cell carcinoma. Metastasis does not occur, though the draining lymph nodes are often reactively enlarged. Treatment consists of wide local excision.

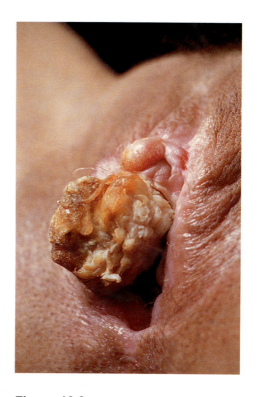

Figure 10.9
Verrucous carcinoma. This huge tumour grew on a 60-year-old woman over a period of a few months. In her case lichen sclerosus was also present.

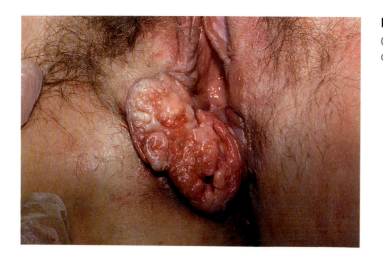

Figure 10.10
Cauliflower-like verrucous carcinoma of Buschke–Löwenstein.

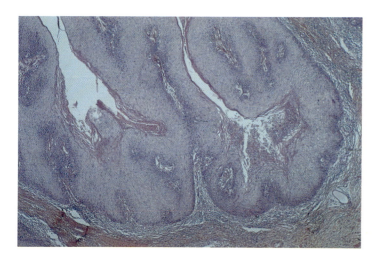

(a)

Figure 10.11
Biopsy must be a deep
surgical specimen.
(a) Low-power morphology,
with well-defined lobes of
epithelium proliferating deep
into the dermis. (b) This is
another example showing the
pale clear keratinocytes which
are characteristic of verrucous
carcinoma.

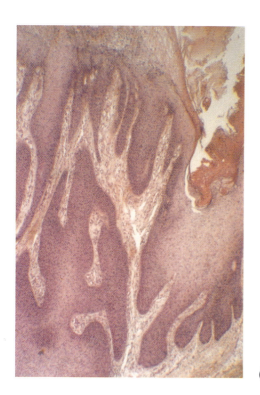

(b)

Paget's disease of the vulva (intra-epidermal adenocarcinoma)

This rare disease affects older women and usually presents as a non-healing red, crusted and eroded plaque, often of surprisingly long standing. Unlike Paget's disease of the nipple, association with underlying adenocarcinoma is rare (about 10%). However, association with distant carcinomas, including uterus, renal tract, gastrointestinal tract and breasts, is more frequent.

Management

1   A clinical history should be taken to uncover suggestions of underlying malignancy. Perianal Paget's disease necessitates colonoscopy. In cases with vulval lesions, there should be investigation of the renal tract, lower abdominal ultrasound, and careful breast and vaginal examination.
2   Management is by local excision and laser treatment of clinically evident disease. Heroic surgery should no longer be considered, as the disease is multifocal and recurrences can be dealt with as they occur, with simple local measures.
3   The patient should be followed up and any recurrences treated by laser or excision.
4   Topical corticosteroids can help pruritus.

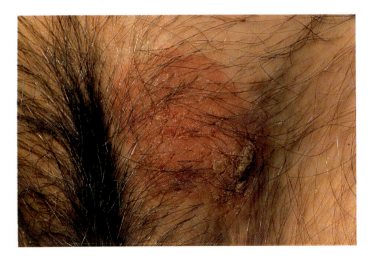

Figure 10.12
Paget's disease of the pubic skin. This well-demarcated red, eroded plaque failed to heal with topical corticosteroids. Biopsy showed this to be Paget's disease.

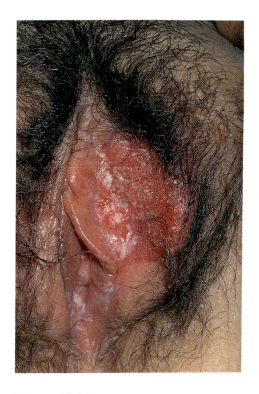

Figure 10.13

Paget's disease. This pruritic lesion in the left interlabial sulcus is another example.

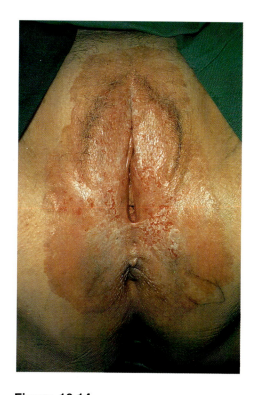

Figure 10.14

Paget's disease. Extensive spread can occur in neglected cases. Note the crisp demarcation and multiple erosions, bearing witness to the pruritic nature of the condition.

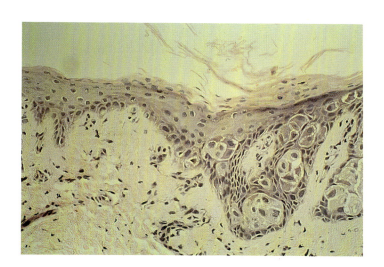

Figure 10.15

Histology of Paget's disease. This is a typical histological picture with nests of large clear cells (which are PAS and alcian blue positive) in the lower epidermis (H & E, ×83).

Langerhans' cell histiocytosis

This histiocytic proliferation can present with haemorrhagic papular, nodular or ulcerative lesions of the anogenital skin. Flexural and mucosal sites are often involved. Histology shows nests of histiocytes in the epidermis, invading the dermis, and usually mixed with eosinophils. Such cells are CD1-positive and ultrastructurally show 'tennis-racket' like inclusion bodies characteristic of Langerhans' cells. Such localized lesions are usually part of a more widespread involvement, which can affect lung, bones, or hypophysis. Lesions can resolve spontaneously. Persistent disease may respond to local or systemic cytotoxics as required.

Management
1 All patients should be referred to specialist centres for evaluation and treatment.
2 Local or systemic cytotoxic treatment is required.

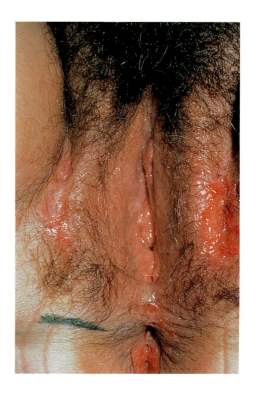

Figure 10.16

Langerhans' cell histiocytosis showing ulcerated haemorrhagic plaques.

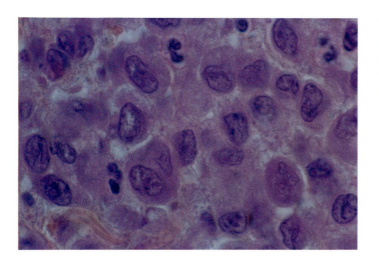

Figure 10.17

Histology of Langerhans' cell histiocytosis. There is widespread dermal invasion with histiocytes (H & E, ×300).

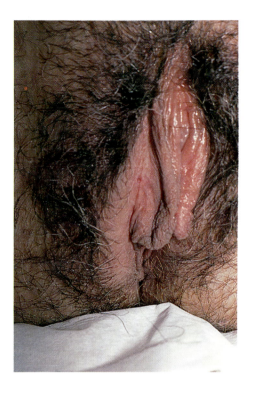

Figure 10.18

Langerhans' cell histiocytosis. Some 8 years before this photograph was taken, the patient, then aged 32, was diagnosed as having diabetes insipidus. A small scattering of dark red papules appeared on the skin but the histology was uncertain and only biopsy of this papular erosive lesion of the vulva confirmed the diagnosis of Langerhans' cell histiocytosis.

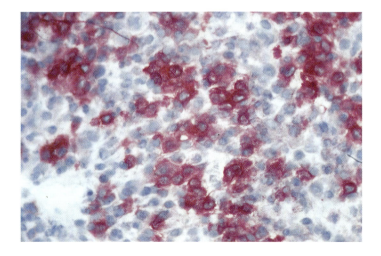

Figure 10.19

Histology of Langerhans' cell histiocytosis, showing positive alkaline phosphatase immuno-staining with a monoclonal-CD1 antibody (×40).

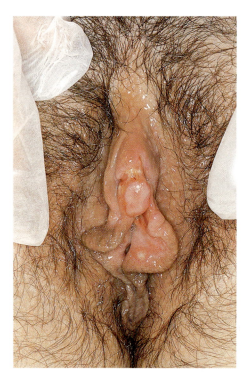

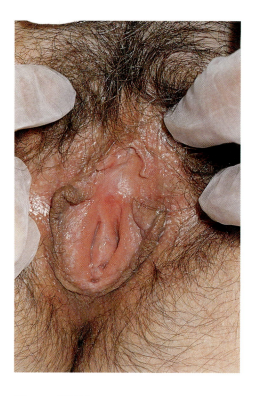

Figure 10.20
Langerhan's cell histiocytosis in a 26-year-old
woman, showing peri-clitoral tumour and
ulceration.

Figure 10.21
The same patient 5 months later, showing
healing following systemic and topical
corticosteroid treatment.

Basal cell carcinoma

Basal cell carcinomas (rodent ulcers) only occur where there are pilosebaceous units. (They are thought to derive from the epithelia of the pilar orifice.) They grow slowly and may be nodular and have a characteristic pearly edge, or more rarely, be flat and atrophic. Older lesions ulcerate and bleed. Most lesions are greyish in colour with prominent telangiectasia but some can become pigmented. They are rare in vulval skin and usually occur after the age of 50.

Management

Local surgical excision, and not vulvectomy, is the treatment of choice. Histological confirmation of clearance is necessary.

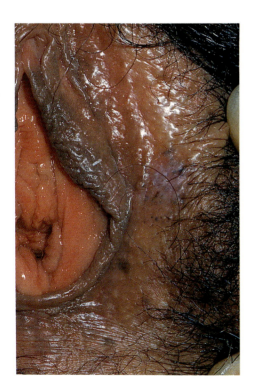

Figure 10.22

Basal cell carcinoma in a 50-year-old woman. Note the well-demarcated pearly edge and flecks of pigmentation.

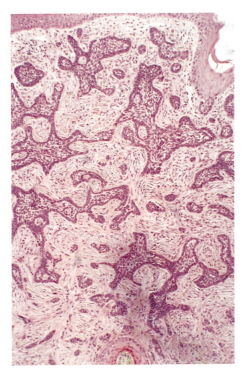
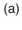

(a)

Figure 10.23
Histology of vulval basal cell carcinoma. (a) There is 'basaloid' proliferation with peripheral pallisading. Clefts form between these and the specialized surrounding stroma (H & E, ×40).

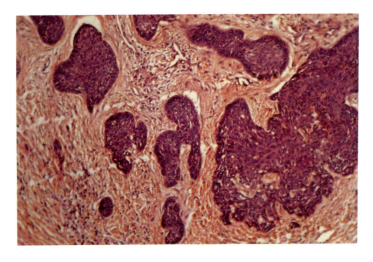

(b)

(b) Enlargement of the same specimen (H & E, ×83).

Malignant melanoma

These tumours represent 5% of all malignancies in the vulva. Although the incidence of malignant melanoma in non-genital skin is increasing at an alarming rate, there is no evidence to suggest that this is the case for vulval skin. This is further evidence for the widely held belief that sunlight is the major environmental aetiological factor for malignant melanoma. The most common site in women is the calf, and the vulval clinic can provide an opportunity for checking this area. Any patient with vulval malignant melanoma should have her *whole* skin examined. Prognosis is determined by depth of invasion.

The experience at Hôpital Tarnier in central Paris over 10 years (1979–1989), may put the incidence of malignant melanoma into perspective: non-genital malignant melanomas, 490 patients; vulval melanomas, 10 patients.

As in non-genital skin, the majority of malignant melanomas are of the superficial spreading type (70%), the remaining 30% being nodular lesions carrying a worse prognosis.

All localized pigmented lesions of the vulva should be subjected to biopsy.

The prognosis of malignant melanoma of the vulva is determined by the Breslow thickness: this is the measurement to the deepest intruding cell from the granular layer in the thickest block of the tumour.

Management

1   Management of malignant melanoma of the vulva is the same as for lesions elsewhere in the body, being determined by the Breslow thickness. Early surgery is curative.
2   Local excision is the treatment of choice. Extensive surgery does not improve prognosis.
3   Extensive disease should probably be managed by conservative means rather than aggressive local surgery, with its consequent discomfort and subsequent problems with micturition and lymphatic drainage.

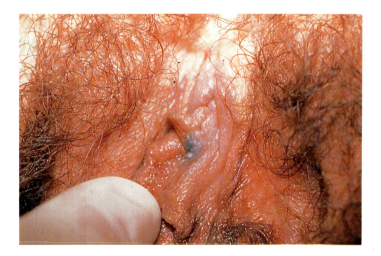

Figure 10.24

Superficial spreading malignant melanoma. There is a small lesion on the labia minora, which is the common vulval site for this tumour.

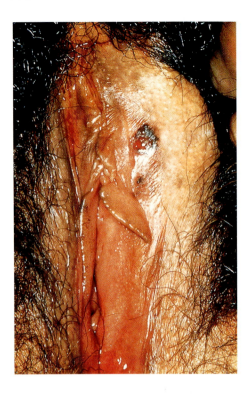

Figure 10.25
Malignant melanoma at one o'clock.

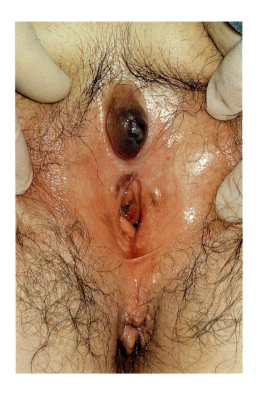

Figure 10.26
Malignant melanoma above the clitoris. Note
the pigment spillage into the surrounding skin.

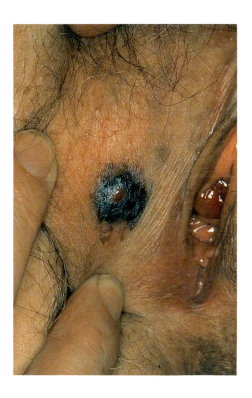

Figure 10.27
Malignant melanoma—nodular type lesion. This carries a poor prognosis because of its depth.

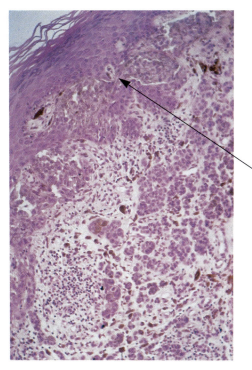

Figure 10.28
Malignant melanoma. Histology of atypical melanocytic proliferation within the epidermis with pagetoid upward migration. Note the atypical melanocytes in the dermis, surrounded by inflammatory cells (H & E, ×40).

Migrating atypical melanocyte
(Pagetoid appearance)

11 Pigmented lesions

Benign melanocytic lesions

Pigmented lesions include compound naevi, intradermal naevi, junctional naevi, blue naevi and lentigo simplex. They are uncommon. Differentiation of these from early malignant lesions is even more difficult than on non-genital skin as most patients cannot give a reliable history of duration or change. Probably the best policy is to remove all such lesions, not because they are more likely to undergo malignant change, but because they are in a hidden site and change might not be easily observed. An isolated pigmented lesion on the vulva, with no definite history of previous inflammation, should be biopsied.

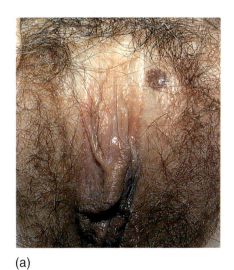

(a)

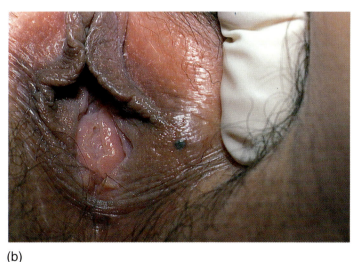

(b)

Figure 11.1
(a) Benign compound naevus; (b) blue naevus.

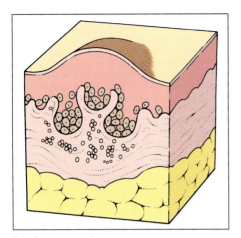

(a) Compound naevus

Figure 11.2
Various types of pigmented lesions.

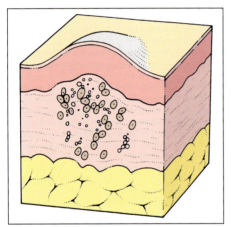

(b) Intradermal naevus

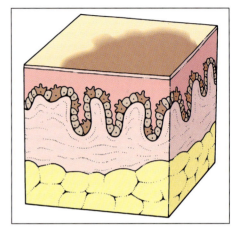

(d) Lentigo simplex

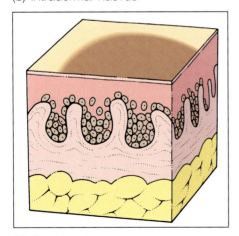

(c) Junctional naevus

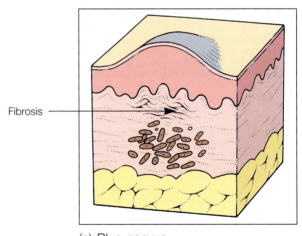

(e) Blue naevus

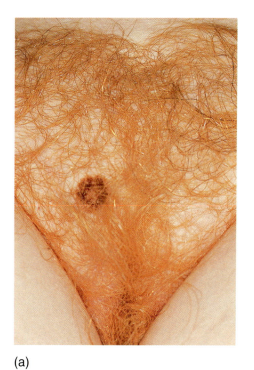

(a)

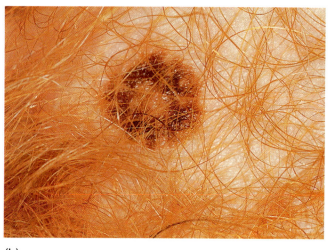

(b)

Figure 11.3

(a) Compound naevus situated on the mons pubis. (b) Closer view of the compound naevus of (a)

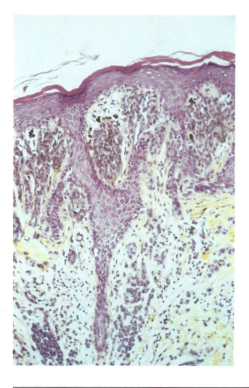

Figure 11.4

Histology of compound naevus. There are nests of pigmented naevus cells in the dermis and pigmentary incontinence. Note the proliferation of junctional melanocytic cells (H & E, ×40).

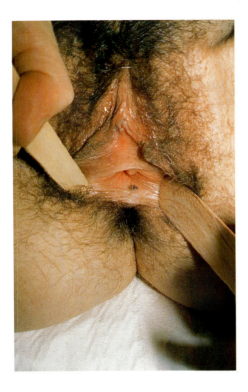

Figure 11.5
Lentigo simplex. Lentigines can be multiple.

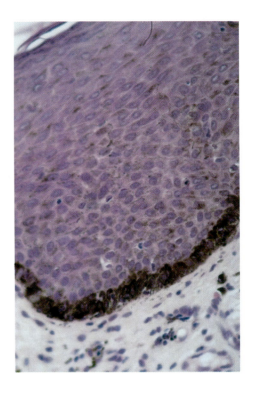

Figure 11.6
Histology of lentigo simplex. This is the characteristic histology, with hyperpigmentation of the basal area with discrete melanocytic proliferation (H & E, ×40).

Other pigmented lesions

All types of inflammation, but especially destructive ones such as lichen sclerosus or lichen planus, can lead to areas of pigmentation. This is called post-inflammatory hyperpigmentation and may persist for months or even years. Usually, the evidence of the inflammation will still be present to help with the diagnosis and sometimes the history will be reliable. Such areas of pigmentation are usually multiple and grouped. If there is any doubt about the source of pigmentation, biopsy should be performed, and this is particularly the case for isolated areas of pigmentation.

In idiopathic acquired pigmentation (of Laugier) patients usually have multiple macular areas of hyperpigmentation on the vulva with no history of antecedent inflammation. At present the condition is thought to be idiopathic and is poorly understood. Histology shows both dermal pigmentary incontinence and some hyperpigmentation of the basal area without melanocytic proliferation.

Vitiligo, a common autoimmune disorder, often presents symmetrically in periorificial sites, especially around the genitalia.

A proportion of mucous cysts will have a blue coloration. This is an optical effect. Excision is required to determine the histological nature of such a lesion.

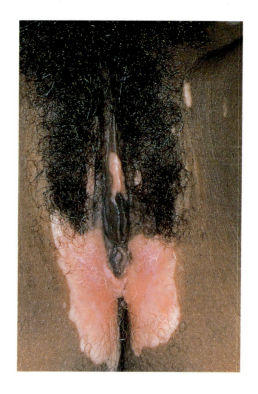

Figure 11.7

Vitiligo —showing stark symmetrical complete depigmentation of genital skin.

Management

1 All localized pigmented lesions of the vulva should be subjected to biopsy (see Figures 2.9–2.11).
2 More diffuse pigmentary change can be sampled by punch biopsy.
3 The histological interpretation of some benign melanocytic proliferations in the vulva can be difficult, and second opinions may be indicated.

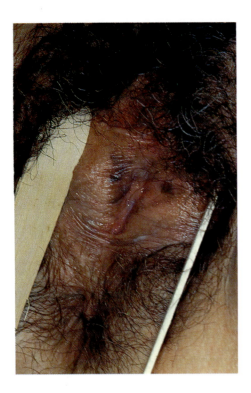

Figure 11.8
Idiopathic acquired pigmentation (of Laugier).

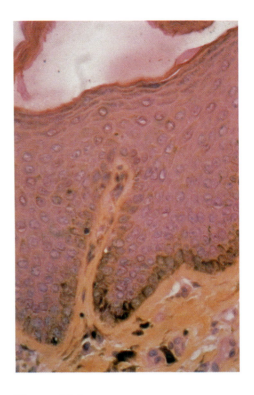

Figure 11.9
Idiopathic acquired pigmentation (of Laugier).
There is hyperpigmentation of the basal layer,
with no proliferation of melanocytes and some
underlying dermal pigmentary incontinence
(H&E, × 40).

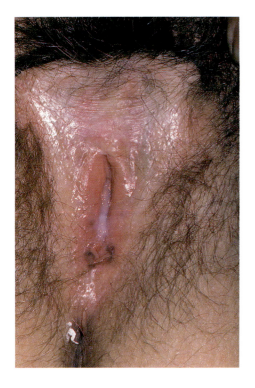

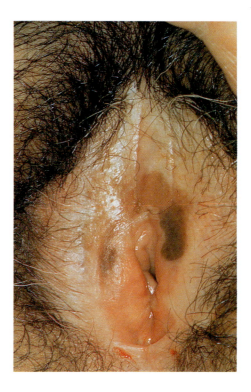

Figure 11.10
Post-inflammatory hyperpigmentation. This
case occurred following lichen planus.

Figure 11.11
Post-inflammatory hyperpigmentation. This
case occurred following lichen sclerosus.

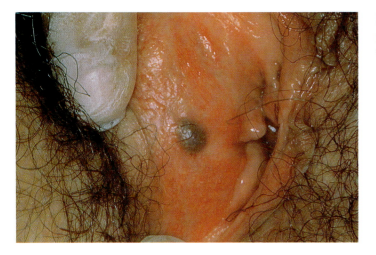

Figure 11.12
Pigmented mucous cyst of the
vestibule.

12 Vulval diseases in childhood

Vulval infections in childhood

There are scant data on the incidence and prevalence of sexually transmitted infections in children and young adolescents. For the individual clinician, the possibility that a child may have acquired a sexually transmitted condition raises several issues of both clinical and forensic management. The possibility of sexual abuse must be considered; however, transmission of infections following sexual abuse must be differentiated from the acquisition of infections by vertical or accidental transmission of the same microbe. For instance, genital herpes simplex virus infection and human papilloma virus infection may both be acquired vertically, and appear in young children.

Several principles must be observed in the management of children with suspected genital infections. It is essential that microbiological tests are properly conducted to achieve the maximum chance of obtaining a diagnosis. This is both for clinical management and medico-legal reasons. It is essential that well-documented and descriptive records are taken of the clinical appearances in children. Of paramount importance in all of this is the maintenance of the highest possible standards of care for the child herself, who must be managed in as sensitive and as carefully controlled way as possible. The number of examinations and invasive tests must be kept to the absolute minimum and continuity of management by one clinician is essential in such cases.

Most STDs of adults have also been reported in children. It is only with better management of suspected cases of child sexual abuse, and the taking of specimens for microbiological examinations, that the true incidence and prevalence of genital infections in children will ever become known. However, the acquisition of such data must be balanced against the need for minimizing the trauma to the child during both investigation and therapy.

Lichen sclerosus

This can present in childhood and is more commonly diagnosed in girls than in boys. One explanation for this is the failure to examine histologically the prepuces of boys circumcised for medical reasons. Phimosis is the most frequent presentation of the disease in young boys.

Constipation is often the presenting history in girls with peri-anal lichen sclerosus because of the painful fissuring associated with this disease (see page 22).

Sexual abuse

In our experience, the vulval clinic is an unlikely place for such patients to present, but the prevalence of sexual abuse may well be under-estimated. It must be considered in children with recurrent discharges or sexually transmitted lesions about the vulva. Warts and molluscum contagiosum are not uncommon infections of flexural sites in children, especially in those with a tendency to atopic dermatitis. The presence of viral warts in vulval or perianal skin should be borne in mind as a possible presentation of child sexual abuse, but such lesions can certainly be acquired non-sexually. Infections that should raise more suspicion are those that are commonly sexually transmitted, such as gonor-rhoea, herpes simplex and chlamydia.

There are no absolute diagnostic signs to establish a diagnosis of child sexual abuse, but abnormal bruising and tears, particularly of the anus and posterior fourchette, should be regarded with suspicion.

Lichen sclerosus in a young girl certainly does occur and, because of the scarring and purpura, may be misinterpreted by the inexperienced as traumatic.

The most appropriate clinician to investigate suspected abuse will depend on local circum-stances, but the experienced and sympathetic paediatrician will usually be the most practised in dealing with these cases. The over-zealous pursuit of such a suspicion can be harmful in itself and can inflict lasting damage on the child or the family.

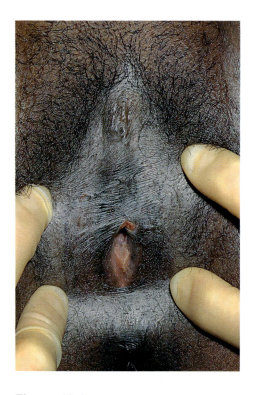

Figure 12.1

This 25-year-old Sudanese woman presented with inability to have intercourse. The clitoris is absent, with gross scarring and narrowing of the introitus with loss of the labia minora.

Female genital mutilation

Female genital mutilation (FGM) is still widely practised in Africa. It is thought by some to reduce sexual desire and ensure chastity and fidelity. There are also strong sociological and aesthetic reasons why the practice exists. More than 100 million women have undergone the procedure worldwide, often performed without anaesthetic on young girls aged 4–12 years of age.

The ritual usually takes place with unsterile instruments. Up to 6 people are needed to hold the child down. Closure of the wound is sometimes achieved using acacia thorns and

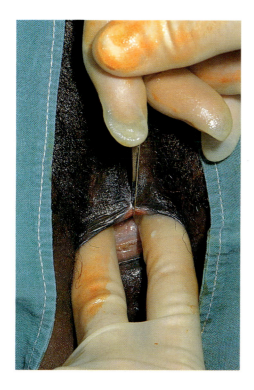

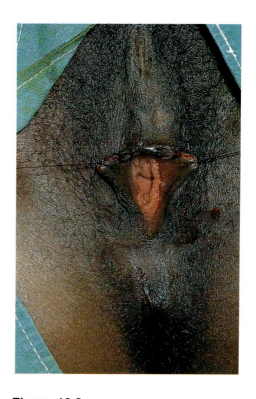

Figure 12.2

Surgery involves a vertical incision through the scar tissue, being careful to avoid the urethra.

Figure 12.3

The edges are sewn up transversely and the introitus is enlarged, exposing the normal hymen. This patient subsequently became pregnant and had a normal vaginal delivery.

horse hair. The girl's legs are usually bound to prevent bleeding and ensure apposition of the tissues, with the application of ash paste as a traditional healing aid.

The practice is illegal in the UK, the USA and in many European countries. However, many African families living abroad arrange for their young girls to return home for 'holidays' at the crucial time prior to puberty. This rite is believed to mark the transition to adulthood.

Types of mutilation

1 Circumcision
This is the removal of the prepuce of the clitoris only (known in Muslim countries as Sunna).

2 Excision
This is the removal of the clitoris and all, or part of, the labia minora.

3 Infibulation
This involves removal of the clitoris, labia minora and at least the anterior two thirds, and often the whole of, the labia majora.

4 Intermediate
This entailes removal of the clitoris and variable amounts of the labia minora and majora.

Epidemiology

The practice is almost universal in Somalia and Djibouti and approximately 90% of girls have undergone female genital mutilation in Ethiopia, Mali, Sudan and Sierra Leone. The distribution of FGM in Africa is given on page 2 of Dorkenoo and Elworthy (1996).

Complications

These include death from infection, haemorrhage and urinary retention. Chronic problems include scarring, keloid and neuroma formation, dysmenorrhoea and urinary symptoms.

Later, problems occur in relation to non-consummation and primitive surgery by the husband is often required before vaginal intercourse can take place.

The most significant complication in pregnancy relates to soft tissue obstruction and tearing of the lower genital tract in labour. If FGM is first diagnosed in pregnancy, gynaecological opinion should be sought prior to delivery as surgery may be required to prevent serious perineal and urethral damage.

These women are often best cared for in a dedicated clinic where other social and cultural factors can be acknowledged. Many African women prefer a female doctor in these circumstances.

There is now a worldwide campaign to change this practice.

13 Psychological aspects of vulval disease

Vulvodynia

This term has been introduced to describe the symptom of pain in the vulva. It is usually chronic pain which is burning or stinging in nature. The classification of vulvodynia is still evolving, but currently there are three main groups recognized:

- Vestibulitis
- Cyclic vulvitis
- Dysaesthetic vulvodynia

The assessment of these patients includes a careful examination of the skin to exclude a dermatosis or infection that may be the cause of their symptoms. A small fissure at the introitus may easily be overlooked, but it may well produce severe symptoms, particularly during intercourse. There is, however, often little to see on inspection of the skin as pain elicits a withdrawal response, so the usual signs of lichenification and excoriation are not seen.

In evaluating these patients it is important to concentrate on the mucosa of the vestibule as this is probably the area most likely to be the origin of a burning sensation. It is also important to test cutaneous sensation over the whole of the perineum.

Vestibulitis

Vestibulitis is the most commonly seen condition in the group collectively called vulvodynia. It is discussed in detail on pages 61–2.

Cyclic vulvitis

The symptoms of cyclic vulvitis are intermittent and related to the menstrual cycle, usually occurring at the time of menstruation. There is often irritation after intercourse, and many of these patients will have marked erythema of the vulva when examined. The aetiology is uncertain, but *Candida albicans* is thought to be implicated as many of these patients do respond to anti-candidal treatment.

Management

Continuous treatment for 4–6 weeks with vaginal anti-candidal agents (e.g. nystatin), or changing the vaginal pH with acetic acid jelly, have been reported to help in selected cases.

Dysaesthetic vulvodynia

Dysaesthesia is defined as the abnormal perception of pain with a stimulus that is normally painless. The pain may be very severe, with the complaint that even underwear next to their skin is intolerable. Patients in this group tend to be older, post-menopausal and have pain that is constant. It is not triggered by intercourse (as in vestibulitis) as the majority of patients are sexually inactive.

There is usually no abnormality on inspection, but attention to sensory testing is an important part of the examination. It is thought that some of these patients do have pudendal neuralgia, and there have been anecdotal reports of abnormalities such as sacral cysts causing this type of pain.

Management

1 Low dose amitriptyline, starting at 10 mg a night and increasing by 10 mg a night each week, is tried until 70 mg a night is reached. Amitriptyline is used because of its central effect on pain although, as many of these patients are clinically depressed, the antidepressant effect is also important. It is argued that the vulvodynia is a symptom of depression, which is the primary diagnosis, however, it is also well recognized that chronic pain leads to secondary depression. Doxepin or fluoxetine may be used if amitriptyline is not tolerated. It is important to supervise these drugs carefully as the majority of patients are elderly and more likely to have cardiac disease, with a higher risk of cardiac side-effects.

2 These patients should have routine ECGs before and during treatment.

3 Carbamazepine, widely used for trigeminal neuralgia, may similarly help with dysaesthetic vulvodynia. Monitoring of the patients' full blood count is important as, rarely, carbamazepine can cause agranulocytosis and aplastic anaemia.

4 Pudendal nerve blocks are not a particularly successful therapy, but newer modalities of treatment are constantly evolving.

5 Pain clinics are becoming a widely available service, and referral of patients with vulvodynia would be appropriate.

6 Patients who fail to respond to any treatment should be assessed to exclude underlying psychopathology.

Appendix I

Plastic repair of the vulva

The vulval architecture can be much changed by disease or the trauma of childbirth. Such alterations can be uncomfortable and may cause dyspareunia.

Simple surgical correction can be effective. (See also pages 123–124).

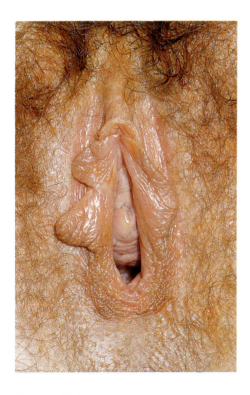

Figure AI.1
Right labial tear following spontaneous vaginal delivery. Patient complained of dyspareunia.

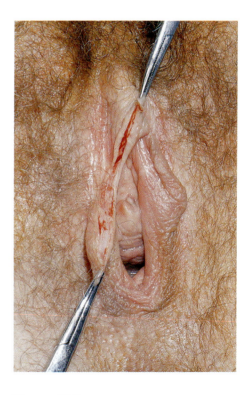

Figure AI.2
Operative view showing excision of inner faces of tear prior to closure.

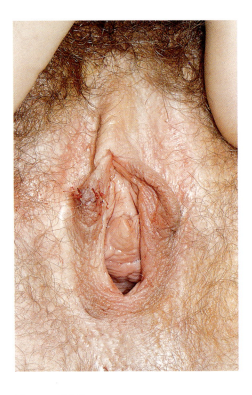

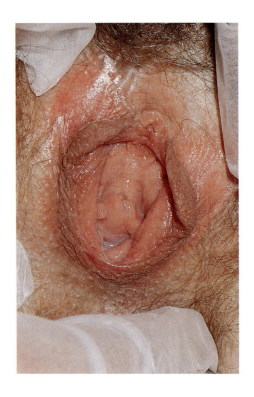

Figure AI.3
After reconstruction.

Figure AI.4
Appearances at eight-week follow-up with
good cosmetic and functional result.

Appendix II

Aqueous cream BP

This is most often dispensed in large 500 g tubs, but 50 or 100 g tubes are much to be preferred on grounds of hygiene and convenience. The patient should be instructed to use this in place of soap for washing since it is less irritating. It is best applied directly to the whole anogenital area *before* bathing or showering. The cream should be gently but completely rinsed off with the hands or a flannel.

Potassium permanganate solutions for soaks, wet dressings and baths

Potassium permanganate solutions can be used as cleansing applications for wet dressings and for soothing soaks. The solution to be used should be freshly prepared. It can be made up from potassium permanganate crystals, a concentrated (1–2%) solution and from commercially available tablets for dilution (Permitabs—Bioglan). The solution is antiseptic, destroying bacteria, fungi, viruses and yeasts. It

is particularly effective in treating acute weeping flexural intertrigo, dissolving away the crusts and scabs that provide a haven for secondary infecting organisms. Sore, inflamed, weeping areas of skin can be much soothed and dried by 10-minute soaks, repeated two to three times daily if necessary. This astringent drying effect, so helpful in acute inflammation and erosions, can be counterproductive if continued too long, leading to over-drying and cracking. Dry, scaly, inflamed areas, such as chronic lichenified eczema or psoriasis, are better cleansed with aqueous cream BP (see above).

Preparation of solution

It is best to make up a concentrated deep purple solution in an old jug first. Either one 400 mg tablet (Permitabs) can be dissolved in one pint of water, or a few crystals or drops of a concentrated 1% solution can be added to the same amount of water, this solution is then used further diluted. To minimize staining of baths, basins and bidets, it is best to fill these first with the required amount of water and then add small quantities from the jug to produce a light pink colour—'vin rosé' and not 'red wine' colour.

Use of potassium permanganate solution

Soak for about 10 minutes in the bath or bidet, or apply a dressing soaked in the solution, for 10 minutes.

Potassium permanganate soaks can stain the nails brown, and this takes several weeks to shed from the surface naturally. Staining can be minimized by painting the nails first with nail varnish or applying a little Vaseline over the nails.

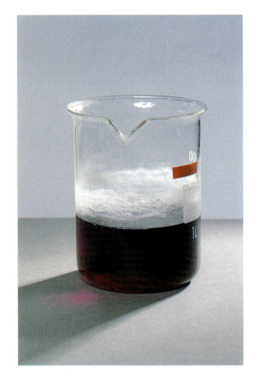

Figure 1
1% potassium permanganate solution.

Figure 2
Potassium permanganate tablets.

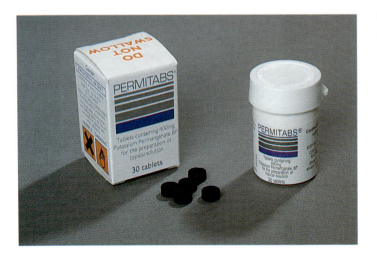

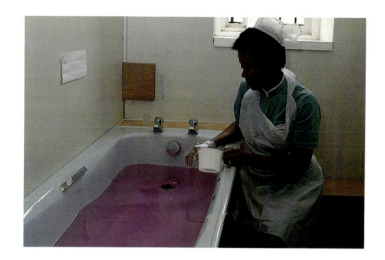

Figure 3
Potassium permanganate bath.

Appendix III

Topical corticosteroids

Hydrocortisone was discovered in the 1950s, and there have been many new and more potent corticosteroids introduced since then. For convenience, they can be graded into four potencies, Grade I being the strongest:

- Grade I—very potent
- Grade II—potent
- Grade III—moderately potent
- Grade IV—mild

It is probably best to become acquainted with one example from each grade. It is also important to know tube size and to instruct patients on exactly *how much* and where the corticosteroid is to be applied. We have found that apparent 'unresponsiveness' to topical corticosteroids has on occasions been due to incorrect usage. Half a gram approximately covers the fingertip and is usually adequate to treat the affected areas, remembering that the vulva is an occluded site.

When recording in notes, or when giving instructions, it is important to record the group as well as the name, for example 'a Grade II steroid was prescribed, Betnovate ointment, 30 g—this must last the full 2 months until the next visit'.

The table opposite records some popular examples of different potencies of commercially available topical corticosteroid preparations and their trade names in different countries.

N.B. Topical corticosteroids sold in the U.K. are not licensed for use in the genital and peri-anal areas and information to this effect may be contained in the packaging. This issue must be carefully discussed with the patient, and clear instructions given on how to use the product safely.

Examples of proprietary products

Grade	Corticosteroid preparation	UK	France	Italy	Germany	Spain	USA
I	Clobetasol propionate	Dermovate	Dermoval	Clobesol	Dermoxin	Clobate	Temovate
II	Betamethasone dipropionate	Diprosone	Diprolene	Diprosone	Diprosone	Diproderm	Diprosone
	Betamethasone 17 valerate	Betnovate	Betneval	Ecoval-70	Betnesol	Betnovate	Valisone Betatrex
	Beclomethasone dipropionate	Propaderm	–	Propaderm	–	–	–
	Fluticasone propionate	Cutivate	–	–	Flutivate	–	Cutivate
	Hydrocortisone butyrate	Locoid	Locoid	Locoid	Alfason	–	Locoid
	Fluocinolone acetonide	Synalar	Synalar	–	–	Synalar	–
	Mometasone furoate	Elocon	–	Elocon Crema	Ecural	Elocom	Elocon
	Triamcinolone acetonide	Adcortyl	Kenacort-A	Kanacort	Volon-A	–	Kenalog Aristocort
III	Clobetasone butyrate	Eumovate	–	Eumovate	Emovate	Emovate	–
	Alclometasone dipropionate	Modrasone	Aclosone	Legaderm	Delonal	Aclodal	Aclovate
IV	Hydrocortisone	Efcortelan	Hydrocortisone Astier	Algicortif Dermacoral	Hydrocortisone Wolff	Crema-Transcotanea – Asti	Cortdome Eldecort Dermacort

Appendix IV

Patient information leaflet (used by authors)

Vulval dermatoses

Lichen sclerosus

This is an inflammation of the skin of unknown cause. It can occur anywhere on the body but most commonly it affects the skin surrounding the vulva and anus. It is often seen at the time of the menopause or before puberty but can occur at any age. The main symptom is itch. In long-standing disease there may be an alteration of the normal anatomy of the vulva. The clitoris becomes buried under the skin and the labia minora may be lost. The entry to the vagina may become narrowed resulting in difficult and painful intercourse. In children the skin around the anus may crack which causes painful defaecation and can lead to constipation. In young boys the foreskin can become tight and cannot be drawn back. Sometimes there is a family history of this skin disease and there is often a family history of other autoimmune disease, such as thyroid gland problems.

Lichen planus

This is also an inflammatory skin condition which can occur anywhere on the skin, but in some individuals it will affect mainly the mucous membranes in the mouth and genital area. It may have changes that are similar to lichen sclerosus but more often it is red and eroded. The main symptom is pain. The areas that are affected are the inner aspects of the vulva, that is the vestibule and the vagina. If the mouth is involved it is usually the gums, inner cheeks or tongue.

Investigations

You will probably need a skin biopsy, that is, a small piece of skin will be cut out. This will be done under a local anaesthetic so it will be painless. You may also have to have a blood test to exclude thyroid gland problems.

Treatment

It is important to stop using all soap and bubble-baths and to use a soap substitute, for example aqueous cream. The most successful treatment is a steroid ointment which is used once a day initially, usually at night. A 30 g tube will last you at least three months, and is quite safe. If you are pregnant or intend to get pregnant, let your doctor know.

Follow up

Once your condition is controlled you will need to have an annual check up, as *rarely* a skin cancer can develop on long-standing chronic inflammation. If you do develop an ulcer or small growth that does not respond to treatment after a month, you must consult your doctor without further delay.

Treatment instructions for lichen sclerosus and lichen planus

You will have been prescribed Dermovate ointment or Propaderm ointment (cream is usually avoided except in certain individual cases).

First month: Once at night, apply a thin layer of the ointment to the affected areas, not forgetting the skin around the anus if this is involved too.

Second month: Apply on alternate nights.

Third month: Apply twice a week.

Maintenance

After this time, you should only need to use your ointment once a week or once a fortnight. If your symptoms return, increase to the number of applications that did control them: for example, if your problems return when you are using the ointment on alternate nights, restart nightly applications.

Quantity

A small amount of any substance put on the skin can be absorbed so it is important to keep within the recommended amounts. The 30 g tube that has been dispensed should last you two or three months. If you do get further supplies please keep a record of the amount you use.

Side effects

There may a burning sensation when you first apply the treatment, but this usually disappears within ten minutes. If the burning persists and is severe, stop using the ointment, as you may be sensitive to one of its components. You should then change to the other ointment listed above.

Follow up

Normally you will be reviewed after your first eight weeks of treatment and then as required. Once your skin condition is stable, you will only have to be seen once every six months or yearly.

Lichen sclerosus in children

Lichen sclerosus is an inflammation of the skin which occurs without a known cause. It is not an infection and it cannot therefore be caught from another person or passed on to someone else. It is associated with other autoimmune diseases such as vitiligo (loss of skin pigment) and alopecia (loss of scalp or body hair). In adult women it is most commonly associated with thyroid gland problems. There is often a history in the family of one of these disorders, so it is believed that lichen sclerosus is related to one's genetic make-up. The commonest area to be affected is the genital skin, although in a few children it can occur on the skin in other areas, particularly the back.

In boys, lichen sclerosus usually causes inflammation and tightening of the foreskin which may be severe enough to require a circumcision, usually around the ages of 6–10. In males, lichen sclerosus very rarely, if ever, spreads to the skin surrounding the anus.

In girls, lichen sclerosus may also involve the skin surrounding the vulva or anus. The commonest symptoms include itch, constipation because of painful cracks in the skin around the anus or pain on passing urine. The skin initially shows inflammation but later becomes white, shiny and crinkly.

The treatment is a strong steroid ointment known as clobetasol proprionate (Dermovate). It has to be used sparingly once at night according to the instructions that the doctor has given you and it is important for you to record the total amount of ointment used. A tube of the steroid ointment normally contains 30 g and this will normally last 6 months to 1 year. The amount that is needed is gradually reduced as the skin disease comes under control.

It may be necessary for your child to be followed up in the clinic for a while, even though the skin responds to the treatment, to make sure that the inflammation does not recur.

Further reading

Adler MW, *ABC of Sexually Transmitted Diseases,* 2nd edn (British Medical Journal Publications: London 1990).

Barter G, Barton S, Gazzard B, *HIV and AIDS: Your Questions Answered* (Churchill Livingstone: London and Edinburgh 1993).

Black MM, McKay M, Braude P, *Colour Atlas and Text of Obstetric and Gynecologic Dermatology* (Mosby-Wolfe: London and Baltimore 1995).

Daniels D, Hillman RJ, Barton SE, Goldmeier D, *Sexually Transmitted Diseases and AIDS* (Springer-Verlag: Berlin 1993).

Dorkenoo E and Elworthy S, *Female Genital Mutilation – Proposals for Change.* (Minority Rights Group International: Place, March 1996)

Friedrich EG, Vulva disease, in *Major Problems in Obstetics and Gynecology*, Vol. 9, 2nd edn (WB Saunders: Philadelphia 1989).

Hewitt J, Pelisse M, Paniel BJ, *Maladies de la vulve* (Medisi–McGraw-Hill: Paris 1987).

Kaufman RH (ed.), Vulvovaginal disease, *Clinical Obstetrics and Gynecology*, Vol. 34, no. 3, Sept. 1991, pp. 581–681 (JB Lippincott: Philadelphia).

Ridley CM, *The Vulva,* 2nd edn (WB Saunders: Philadelphia 1990).

Index

PETECHIAE.